Atlas of Image-Guided Intervention in Regional Anesthesia and Pain Medicine

Atlas of Image-Guided Intervention in Regional Anesthesia and Pain Medicine

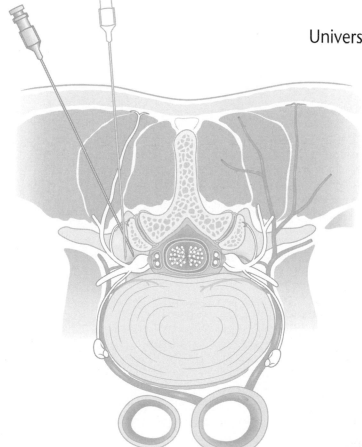

James P. Rathmell, MD

Professor of Anesthesiology
University of Vermont College of Medicine
Director, Center for Pain Medicine
Fletcher Allen Health Care
Burlington, Vermont

Illustrations by

Gary J. Nelson

Medical Illustrator
University of Vermont
College of Medicine
(Retired)

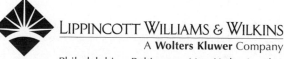

LIPPINCOTT WILLIAMS & WILKINS
A **Wolters Kluwer** Company

Philadelphia • Baltimore • New York • London
Buenos Aires • Hong Kong • Sydney • Tokyo

Acquisitions Editor: Brian Brown
Developmental Editor: Fran Murphy
Project Manager: Nicole Walz
Senior Manufacturing Manager: Ben Rivera
Manufacturing Manager: Angela Panetta
Design Coordinator: Holly Reid McLaughlin
Cover Designer: Armen Kojoyian
Interior Designer: Marie Clifton
Compositor: TechBooks
Printer: Edwards Brothers

© 2006 by LIPPINCOTT WILLIAMS & WILKINS
530 Walnut Street
Philadelphia, PA 19106 USA
LWW.com

Printed in the USA.

Library of Congress Cataloging-in-Publication Data
Rathmell, James P.
   Atlas of image-guided intervention in regional anesthesia and pain medicine / by James P. Rathmell ; illustrations by Gary J. Nelson.
       p. ; cm.
     Includes bibliographical references and index.
     ISBN 0-7817-5181-0 (alk. paper)
   1. Conduction anesthesia—Atlases.   2. Pain—Treatment—Atlases.   3. Pain—Imaging—Atlases.   4. Analgesia—Atlases.   5. Radiography, Medical—Atlases.
I. Title.
   [DNLM: 1. Pain—drug therapy—Atlases.   2. Pain—radiography—Atlases.
3. Anesthesia, Conduction—methods—Atlases.   4. Injections—methods—Atlases.
WL 17 R234a 2006]
RD84.R373 2006 617.9'64075—dc22

2005019157

10 9 8 7 6 5 4 3 2

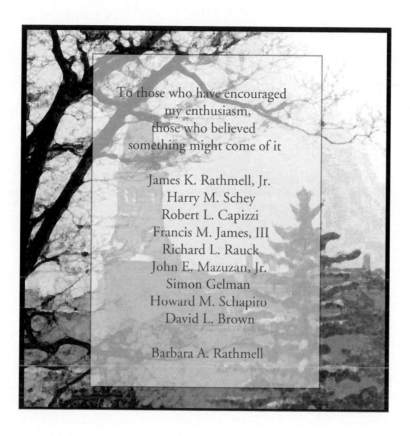

To those who have encouraged
my enthusiasm,
those who believed
something might come of it

James K. Rathmell, Jr.
Harry M. Schey
Robert L. Capizzi
Francis M. James, III
Richard L. Rauck
John E. Mazuzan, Jr.
Simon Gelman
Howard M. Schapiro
David L. Brown

Barbara A. Rathmell

Contents

Preface

During the course of my own training in pain medicine, now well over a decade ago, radiographic guidance was used infrequently—it was reserved for major procedures such as neurolytic celiac plexus block. In the years since my training, I have experienced two forces at work. First, pain practitioners are now being called on to serve as diagnosticians. Patients and referring practitioners expect pain physicians to have familiarity with imaging modalities and their usefulness in diagnosing pain conditions. At the same time, pain practitioners have come to realize the usefulness of radiographic guidance in achieving precise anatomic placement of needles and catheters. Although the evidence supporting the need for routine radiographic guidance is still evolving, the intuitive appeal of this more precise approach has caught firm hold—to the point where the majority of practitioners now perform at least a portion of their injections using fluoroscopic guidance. In some cases, such as with patients with intractable pain associated with metastatic cancer, radiographic guidance has proven invaluable in the planning and implementation of therapy directed toward pain relief. There are numerous excellent atlases for practitioners of regional anesthesia. However, there remains no single, comprehensive and well-illustrated atlas for the pain practitioner that describes both the injection techniques and illustrates the relevant radiographic anatomy. *Atlas of Image-Guided Intervention in Regional Anesthesia and Pain Medicine* is an atlas designed to fill this void.

In 1999, I attended the annual meeting of the American Society of Regional Anesthesia and Pain Medicine (ASRA) in Philadelphia to present a paper on a study I had conducted with a radiologist colleague and a medical student. We examined the distribution of injectate in a series of patients who received epidural steroid injections for radicular pain associated with a new herniated disc. To our surprise, the injectate often spread to the side opposite the disc herniation. In retrospect, this is not at all surprising; if a disc herniation is present on one side, this might well obstruct the flow of fluid through the relatively confined epidural space. The fluid would follow the path of least resistance, spreading preferentially to the contralateral, unaffected side and exiting the contralateral intervertebral foramina. This study and others that emerged at about the same time challenged the conventional wisdom that suspending the steroid in a modest volume was sufficient to consistently produce spread of the injectate to the affected levels, regardless of where the solution was placed within the epidural space. Perhaps the blind loss-of-resistance technique is not the best way to deliver steroid to the site of inflammation.

Using radiographic guidance, we are able to visualize bony structures directly and in real time. We can see the needle within the radiographic field and use simple geometry to guide the needle directly from the skin's surface to its destination. During that same ASRA meeting in 1999, I was introduced to Dr. David Brown, an anesthesiologist and author of several texts on regional anesthesia. He was then Editor-in-Chief of *Regional Anesthesia and Pain Medicine (RAPM)*, and he was in search of a young and enthusiastic Associate Editor to head a new section in *RAPM* on imaging. Although Dr. Brown's well-known text, *An Atlas of Regional Anesthesia*, has sold innumerable copies without anything more than a brief mention of radiographic guidance, he clearly recognized that imaging modalities of all sorts—plain radiography, computed tomography (CT), magnetic resonance imaging, and ultrasound—held untapped potential for advancing the accurate conduct of neural blockade. After a brief discussion, I took the post as Associate Editor, and I have now solicited, written, and reviewed many articles for the Imaging Section in *RAPM*. These articles have helped establish the clear-cut benefit of imaging in the conduct of regional anesthetic techniques in pain medicine, and images from many of the articles are included in this atlas.

The atlas is designed to serve as a practical guide to practitioners who perform (or want to learn how to perform) a wide range of different treatments for acute, chronic, and cancer-related pain with the assistance of radiographic guidance. It is meant to be a useful resource for a range of practitioners. Those already familiar with regional anesthesia but wanting to learn more about the use of radiographic guidance will find the techniques they know illustrated with images encountered when the same techniques are carried out using radiographic guidance. Practitioners already well versed in the use of radiographic imaging will find clinically relevant details, including an overview of each technique, a detailed and illustrated review of the relevant anatomy, technical aspects of each treatment, and a description of the complications associated with these pain treatment modalities.

The atlas begins with an overview of basic techniques for using image guidance to guide needle placement, radiation safety, clinical use of radiographic contrast agents, and the pharmacology of the most common agents used for these injection treatments. The bulk of the atlas is devoted to descriptions of individual techniques. For each technique, concise summaries of common clinical applications, technical details, adverse events, and clinical outcomes are included. Each technique is illustrated using a simple line drawing and the plain x-ray images encountered when the technique is carried out using radiographic guidance. The radiographs are displayed without labels side by side with a detailed overlay on the same image that illustrates the relevant anatomic structures. When published reports suggest that CT might be particularly useful in performing a specific technique (e.g., neurolytic celiac plexus block), details of the CT-guided technique and accompanying CT images are included.

The field of pain medicine suffers from a lack of well-controlled studies to guide our choice of the most effective therapies. Indeed, many of the techniques described in the atlas lack clear evidence to support their efficacy. Even so, the techniques described are in widespread clinical use. I have made every effort to provide a clear summary of the current evidence available supporting the use of each technique, but all too often these data are scant. Precisely because of this lack of outcome data, I have chosen to omit several emerging technologies, including epidural lysis of adhesions and epiduroscopy. The choice of techniques included, although arbitrary, was based on my own perception of those that are performed most commonly. It is my hope that the atlas will help educate and guide practitioners toward a more uniform approach to performing these techniques. With more consistent methodology, we can begin the much-needed work of assembling randomized controlled trials to determine which among these techniques are most useful in aiding those with intractable pain.

JAMES P. RATHMELL, MD
Burlington, Vermont
March 2005

Acknowledgments

This project would not have been possible without the help of many people. First among those who have made this atlas more than a compendium of x-ray images is Gary Nelson, retired medical illustrator at the University of Vermont. I have worked with Gary for many years and was delighted that he was willing to emerge from retirement to complete the illustrations for this book. Gary couples a detailed understanding of anatomy with an absolute attention to detail. When he did not understand a given technique, Gary would venture to my office or to the operating room to see the technique being performed. We would often spend long evening hours by telephone perfecting the details. The results speak for themselves, making this atlas uniquely suited as a practical reference for reviewing the anatomy of each technique as you are about to perform the block.

The images are almost solely from my own practice; my partners in practice, Michael Borrello, Jerry Tarver, Rayden Cody, and Anne Marie Munoz; and our pain fellows during the years the manuscript was in preparation. These fellows, Carlos Pino, Gordon George, Esther Benedetti, Jeffrey Sears, Timothy Lair, Bushra Nauman, Tiffini Lake, Clarence Ivie, and William Megdal, produced many of the radiographs in the atlas in the course of patient care. All my colleagues have helped in choosing the best images and critiquing the manuscript. Dr. Benedetti spent many hours reviewing and sorting through thousands of images to find those best illustrating each technique. My senior research coordinator-turned-medical student, Mark Hoeft, helped keep the project on track, and along the way we have written a number of articles on the subject of image-guided injection. Gary Alsofrom and Jan Gallant, my colleagues in radiology, tolerated the radiologic ignorance of this anesthesiologist, taught me what they could, and provided invaluable assistance at several key points along the way. Suresh Mukerji, Director of Neuroradiology at the University of Michigan, has coauthored a number of articles on imaging in pain medicine and brought his expertise to national lectures on this topic; several of our articles are highlighted in the atlas. Robert Monsey, an orthopedic surgeon and Director of the New England Spine Institute, has been a partner in much of my research. Dr. Monsey helped guide our work in exploring the anatomy of the arterial supply to the spinal cord as it pertains to safe conduct of transforaminal injection of steroids. Mark Manum and John Steidley with Philips Medical Systems offered encouragement and technical expertise in exporting high-quality images and use of digital subtraction technology, and they helped ensure that my discussion and illustration of radiation exposure during c-arm use was sound.

The folks in my academic office, most notably Jude Schofield, Laura Andrews, and Kellie Dutra, made sure I was organized and (reasonably) on time. They helped whenever asked to revise manuscripts, assemble pieces for submission, or field calls from the many folks helping with the project.

The atlas began in 2001, after a discussion with Craig Percy, then an Acquisitions Editor with Lippincott Williams & Wilkins during the annual meeting of the American Society of Anesthesiologists. It took me an additional 2 years and the publication of texts by others on the subject to convince Craig of the value of this atlas, but it was Craig who finally became my ally and a major encouragement for the project. Brian Brown moved into that same role during the latter stages of this project, and I thank him for his frequent checks and cheerleading sessions, which got the manuscript completed. Other key people at Lippincott Williams & Wilkins who brought the project to a close include Fran Murphy, Developmental Editor, who ferried the final submission toward production, and Susan Hermansen, Director of Creative Services, who saw to it that the labeling of the radiographs was made consistent throughout the book.

The encouragement to tackle an entire book on my own came from two people. As Editor-in-Chief of *Regional Anesthesia and Pain Medicine*, David Brown helped me learn how to assemble an article and make it teach something of value to practitioners. This atlas is, quite purposefully, styled after Dr. Brown's *Atlas of Regional Anesthesia*: concise, well illustrated, and meant for everyday use in real clinical practice. I have been involved in many projects with Dr. Brown in more recent years, and he serves as a trusted sounding board and, despite an impossibly busy schedule, always seems to answer the phone whenever I call for advice. My friend and Chair of the Department of Anesthesia at the University of Vermont, Howard Schapiro, has encouraged me through just about every project I have done and is the one who keeps me out of trouble. Dr. Schapiro reminds me that contracts and costs are a reality, and he generously supplied me with time for an unconventional sabbatical, the first in many years in our department, to work on this text.

Finally, and foremost, I thank my family—my wife, Bobbi, and my children, Lauren, James, and Cara. They have simply stared in amazement as I sat day after day, week after week, month after month in my home office—reading, writing, and working with images. During many sunny ski days or beautiful summer weekends, there I was, working away. Thank you all for your tolerance and maybe, just maybe, there will be a real vacation or two in our future.

Foreword

One of the benefits of academic medical practice is interacting with talented and creative physicians. Dr. James P. Rathmell is just such an individual. It has been my distinct pleasure over the last decade to watch Dr. Rathmell, his colleagues at the University of Vermont, and others nationally add new knowledge and techniques to the field of pain medicine, especially those involving image-guided methods. When he asked me to develop a forward to his *Atlas of Image-Guided Intervention in Regional Anesthesia and Pain Medicine,* I was delighted.

For those of you unaware of Dr. Rathmell's background, he is an anesthesiologist who not only is an outstanding educator but also a physician viewed by those knowledgeable as one of our country's leading pain medicine physicians. Dr. Rathmell and I first met while working together on projects for the American Society of Regional Anesthesia and Pain Medicine, while I was editor of our journal, *Regional Anesthesia and Pain Medicine.* After interacting more with Dr. Rathmell I considered the advice from one of my friends from my years in Seattle, Dr. Daniel C. Moore. Dan gave me the advice that as a leader one should always hire people smarter than oneself. Taking this advice to heart, I recognized that Dr. Rathmell was smarter than I was, so I asked him to help with the Society's journal. Reflecting on where real advances in medicine were occurring, it was clear that advances in imaging were driving the largest part of the change, and I wanted our subspecialty to develop more expertise in imaging in regional anesthesia and pain medicine. Thankfully, Dr. Rathmell agreed to help the Journal and developed the imaging section as one of the most frequently read and popular sections of the publication.

As an aside, one of my favorite experiences in interacting with Dr. Rathmell during the early years of our friendship occurred during a meeting of the European Society of Regional Anesthesia held in Barcelona, Spain. During a break in the meeting, Dr. Rathmell and I found time to walk along the harbor. I believe it was at this time that many of the concepts that make this an excellent text were discussed and matured. Additionally, one of the aspects that I still treasure about the harbor walk was Dr. Rathmell's willingness to consider issues even larger than details of image-guided techniques.

Dr. Rathmell has the remarkable ability to blend cutting-edge clinical care with both common sense and creativity. This combination is so rare in academic medicine.

Over the last decade, Dr. Rathmell has also been involved with many of our initiatives to improve pain medicine training across multiple specialties and has been invaluable in developing a unified curriculum for pain medicine physicians entering our field.

In this project, Dr. Rathmell purposely developed an atlas that is designed to provide direct, simple instructions for those completing imaged-guided pain medicine and regional techniques, while underpinning the work with well-developed radiographic aids. After reading and reviewing an advanced version of this work, I know he has succeeded in all his aims. I also believe the illustrator of the book, Mr. Gary Nelson, has succeeded greatly in the very necessary merging of clinical concepts and images in a way that adds tremendous value to this work. Having some experience in merging images and concepts in some of my own books, I am convinced that the partnership between Mr. Nelson and Dr. Rathmell is one for which we should all be thankful.

The first section of this *Atlas* is reason alone to own it. Dr. Rathmell's work in distilling important details of imaging, radiation safety, contrast agents, and drugs used in imaged-guided pain medicine makes this book the single best source for these subjects for pain medicine physicians I've ever read. It is my belief that every physician involved in the clinical care of pain medicine patients needs to read and reread and then go on to fully understanding this first section.

The individual techniques in the other chapters are organized in a clear, standardized fashion: covering first an overview of the technique and then predictably and logically taking the reader through the important anatomy, considerations of patient selection, and patient and fluoroscopic positioning requirements while offering pearls about the technique itself, possible complications, and finally, additional readings that explore unique aspects of the particular image-guided procedure. The predictable sequence makes each chapter effectively stand alone, with the caveat that Section I of the *Atlas* has already been reviewed. Dr. Rathmell's ability to organize is evident in this work, and one of the reasons I suggest that all pain medicine physicians-in-training, and all those involved in caring for patients requiring image-guided techniques, own this book.

Of course, the *Atlas* section on implantable devices is another that alone justifies owning this work. Having watched this part of pain medicine practice mature over my career, I find that Dr. Rathmell's descriptions of implantable techniques are the most straightforward available.

In closing, I want to thank Dr. Rathmell and his family for the investment of time and energy that a project such as this requires. I know that his wife Bobbi and his children all gave up a dear piece of their husband and father while this work was being developed. Finally, I also want to honor all the patients who willingly undergo these techniques and who allow all of us involved in pain medicine to truly "practice medicine" as patients require.

DAVID L. BROWN, MD
Edward Rotan Distinguished Professor
Department of Anesthesiology and Pain Medicine
University of Texas–M.D. Anderson Cancer Center
Houston, Texas

BASIC TECHNIQUES, RADIATION SAFETY, AND PHARMACOLOGY

Basic Techniques for Image-Guided Injection

Patient Positioning and c-Arm Alignment

Throughout this book, suggestions for patient positioning and alignment of the c-arm are illustrated for each type of block (Fig. 1-1). The patient's position is chosen with three factors in mind: safety, access for the block, and patient comfort, in this order of priority. Safety is first. An understanding of the anatomy is paramount, thus the description of each block will begin with a discussion of the relevant regional anatomy. Avoiding critical structures is best accomplished at the outset in planning the approach for neural blockade. A good example is found in the celiac plexus block. Although the rib margins and the vertebral column are easily visualized under fluoroscopy, inferring the position of the abdominal aorta, the diaphragm and pleural reflections, and the adjacent liver, kidney, and spleen is crucial to performing this block successfully and safely. As you review the regional anatomy for each block, it will be apparent that the same target can be approached from many different angles, but often only a single technique is illustrated. The illustrated techniques have been chosen with an eye toward minimizing the risks of the procedure. Although some approaches are actually simpler to perform (e.g., cervical medial branch blocks from a lateral approach), they are best reserved for experienced practitioners because of the inherent dangers in getting confused by the complex radiographic anatomy of the cervical spine. Finally, when all else is equal, position might best be chosen to promote patient comfort. Indeed, most patients are more comfortable in the supine position, particularly for cervical injections, than in the prone position. Once you understand the anatomy of the target for any given block and the critical structures between the skin's surface and the needle's final destination, you may choose to vary both patient position and alignment of the c-arm to suit your own preferences.

Alignment of the c-arm is illustrated for each block, and the approximate angle of the c-arm is also described within the text. The accepted convention is to describe the position and angle of the c-arm according to the direction the x-rays travel from the x-ray source, through the patient, to the image intensifier. To minimize radiation exposure, the x-ray source is typically kept under the x-ray table (see Fig. 2-5). Thus, when the patient is placed prone without angulation of the c-arm, an *anterior-posterior* radiograph is obtained, and when they are place supine, a *posterior-anterior* radiograph results. Lateral movement of the c-arm from the sagittal plane is termed *oblique* angulation. Likewise, when the x-ray path is angled away from the axial plane toward the head, this is termed *cranial* angulation and toward the foot is termed *caudal* angulation.

The Coaxial Technique

Central to using image guidance to facilitate speed, comfort, and accuracy of most injections is an understanding and use of a coaxial technique. The term "coaxial" is used to emphasize that the advancing needle and the x-ray path share a common axis. In this way, the needle tip is advanced from the skin's surface to the final target at a depth with only small changes in the needle's direction. The needle tip and the target are seen at all times. Contrast this with a more traditional means of using surface landmarks to determine the initial site of needle entry through the skin, followed by advancing the needle until it contacts a bony surface. Any adjustments in needle direction require that the needle is withdrawn its entire length before redirection. In the past, radiographic guidance was used, if at all, only to confirm the needle's final position.

To illustrate the coaxial technique, intra-articular lumbar facet injection is shown in Figure 1-1. The patient is positioned prone. The lumbar facet joint to be injected is brought into clear view by moving the c-arm to align the x-ray path with the axis of the joint (see Fig. 1-1A). Once the facet joint is seen clearly, a radiopaque marker is placed on the skin's surface until it overlies the target joint (see

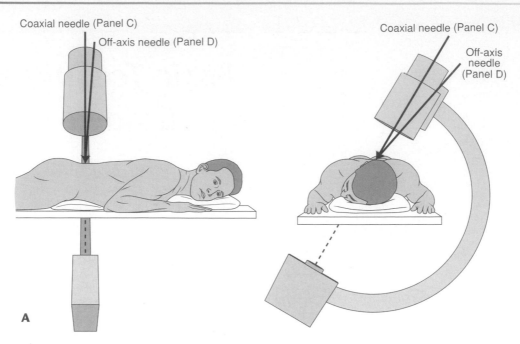

Figure 1-1.
The coaxial technique for needle placement. **A:** Patient position and axis of the c-arm are shown for coaxial intra-articular left lumbar facet injection. The axis of the needle shown in panel C (coaxial) and panel D (off-axis) are shown.

Fig. 1-1B). In this way, the area of skin directly overlying the target along the x-ray axis is identified. The skin and subcutaneous tissues are then anesthetized directly under the tip of the surface marker using a small amount of local anesthetic. The needle is inserted a short distance until it is seated in the subcutaneous tissues overlying the target. The angle of the needle should be adjusted until it is roughly parallel to the x-ray axis. This initial adjustment is performed without taking any radiographs—a glance at the axis of the c-arm image intensifier in comparison to the axis of the needle is all that is needed to bring them into rough alignment during initial needle placement. The needle should remain quite superficial until it is well aligned with the x-ray beam (see Fig. 1-1C). The needle is perfectly aligned with the x-ray beam when the hub of the needle is superimposed on the tip and appears as a radiolucent circle. Only after it is well aligned should the needle be advanced any deeper. Some examples of common difficulties with initial needle placement are shown: Figure 1-1D illustrates poor needle alignment, and Figure 1-1E shows the needle in good coaxial alignment, but not overlying the target. As long as the needle is directed toward the final target, needle advancement continues until the target is reached. If the needle is coaxial but does not lie over the final target, the needle should be removed and replaced over the target. Small changes in needle direction from coaxial can be accomplished easily; large deviations inevitably lead to multiple needle passes to steer the needle to its final destination.

Needles

The most common needle used for image-guided injection is the 22-gauge, 3.5-inch (approximately 10 cm), Quincke spinal needle (Fig. 1-2). This length is suitable for all but the deepest injections. The Quincke point is sharp and advances easily through most tissues. The 22-gauge diameter is a reasonable compromise between needle diameter and stiffness. Although smaller diameter needles produce slightly less pain during placement, they lack stiffness and tend to bend easily.

Several manufacturers now produce blunt tip or rounded tip needles (Fig. 1-3), with the idea that the blunt tip is less likely to penetrate nerves or arteries during placement. Most needles are also available with curved tips placed by the manufacturer (see Fig. 1-3) that allow the needle to be "steered" as it is advanced. Alternately, a curve can easily be placed at the tip of most straight needles by the operator at the time of use.

The most common needle used for performing epidural injection using the loss-of-resistance technique via an interlaminar route is the Touhy needle (Fig. 1-4). Touhy needles are manufactured with a curve in the tip of the needle that directs the distal orifice of the needle nearly perpendicular to the axis of the needle's shaft. The needle was designed to direct a catheter advanced through the needle along the axis of the epidural space, parallel to the dura mater. The Touhy needle remains useful for single-shot epidural techniques, catheter placement, and epidural spinal cord electrode

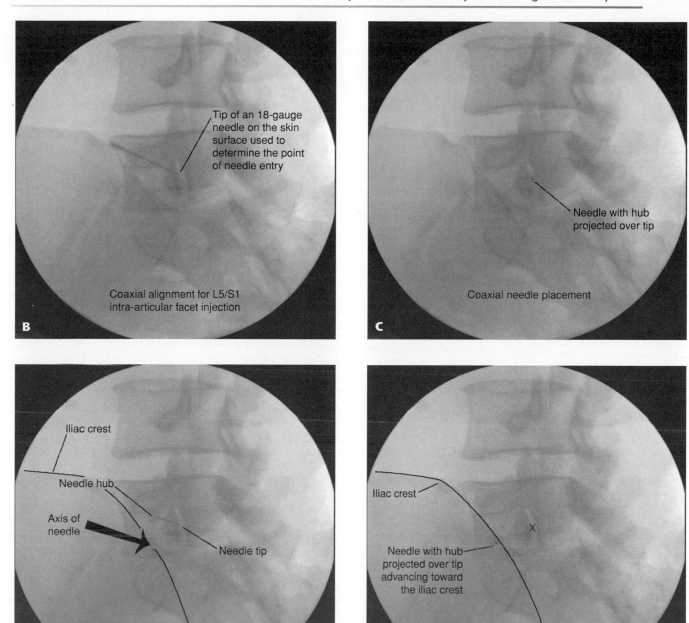

Figure 1-1. *(Continued)*
B: The L5/S1 facet joint is shown with the articular surfaces in good alignment. An 18-gauge needle has been placed on the skin surface overlying the target to determine the point to anesthetize the skin. **C:** A coaxial needle shown in good position over the L5/S1 facet joint. The hub of the needle lies directly over the tip of the needle. **D:** The needle is approaching the L5/S1 facet joint off axis from the x-ray beam, from lateral to medial. **E:** The needle is entering in good coaxial alignment but does not overly the target (X) of the L5/S1 facet joint.

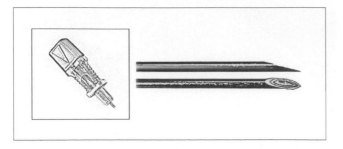

Figure 1-2.
Quincke needle. The 22-gauge, 3.5-inch Quincke spinal needle is the most common needle used by many practitioners for image-guided injection. The Quincke needle has a sharp bevel that advances easily through tissue planes. Most manufacturers produce a needle with a central stylette that has a small notch in the hub. The notch lies on the same side as the needle's bevel face and can be used to determine the direction of the bevel as the needle is advanced.

placement. Touhy needles are available in a range of sizes, the most common being 18- and 20-gauge diameter and 8 cm in length.

Changing the Direction of an Advancing Needle

With use of a precise coaxial technique, only small changes in needle direction are needed to steer the needle to the final destination. The most precise needle placement with the fewest and smallest changes in direction is best accomplished with the use of a precise coaxial technique and a simple beveled needle *without* any additional bend placed near the tip.

To illustrate the techniques used to position a needle, a straight 22-gauge, 3.5-inch spinal needle is shown in

Figure 1-5. Most manufacturers have placed a notch in the hub of the needle with a lock-and-key design. The notch serves to lock the stylette of the needle in position, and it also indicates the direction that the needle's bevel is facing. Beveled needles will naturally veer slightly away from the face of the bevel as they advance through tissue (Fig. 1-6); thus, the bevel should be turned to face away from the direction the operator wants the needle tip to move as it is advanced. However, the magnitude of deviation of a straight, bevel-tip needle is quite small, typically causing the needle tip to veer only a few millimeters as it advances. More drastic changes in needle direction are best accomplished by simply realigning the needle while it is in the superficial tissues (see Fig. 1-5A). Once the needle is seated within the tissues at a depth beyond the first few centimeters, dramatic changes in needle direction are difficult to accomplish, and most often require that the needle be retracted to a more superficial level and redirected. One simple means of "steering" a needle that has been seated more deeply is to grasp the needle at the point where it enters the skin with one hand and at the needle's hub with the other hand. By anchoring the needle's shaft at the midpoint and moving the midshaft in a direction opposite the direction the hub is moved, an arc is created along the shaft of the needle (see Fig. 1-5B), and the needle can be effectively steered in any direction desired. Avoid bending the needle so aggressively that it does not return to a straight line when the needle is released. Overly aggressive bending seldom results in more effective steering and ultimately results in a distorted, misshapen needle that is difficult or impossible to direct any further. Extreme and repeated bending of the needle can also lead to fracture of the needle along the shaft.

Some practitioners advocate creating a small bend several millimeters proximal to the tip of the needle. Indeed, many manufacturers market needles with "curved" or "angled" tips for just this purpose. This small curve causes

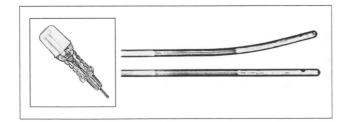

Figure 1-3.
Blunt nerve block needle. Some manufacturers produce blunt-tip needles with the idea that the rounded needle tip will be less likely to penetrate nerves or vascular structures. Most needles are supplied either straight or with a curved tip to facilitate redirection of the needle as it is advanced.

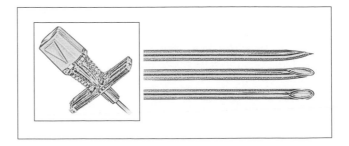

Figure 1-4.
Touhy epidural needle. The Touhy needle is among the most common needles for interlaminar epidural injection using a loss-of-resistance technique. The needle's orifice is aligned nearly perpendicular to the shaft to direct a catheter threaded through the needle along the plane of the epidural space.

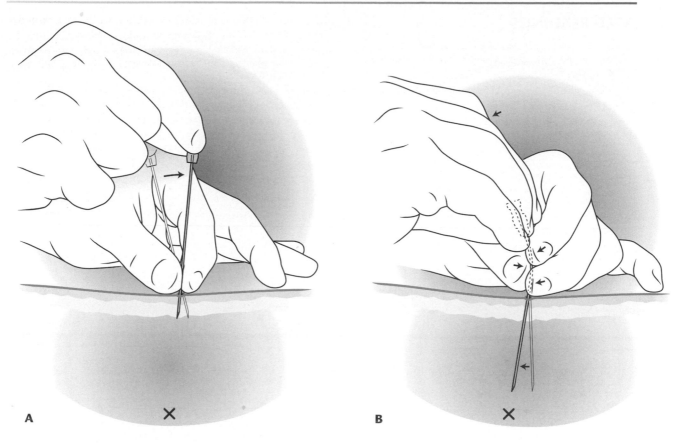

A   X   B   X

Figure 1-5.

Changing the direction of an advancing needle. **A:** Changing the needle direction when the needle tip remains superficial is accomplished by simply changing the axis of the straight needle. The tip will move opposite to the direction of the hub and can be aligned with the desired target (X) before advancing the needle any further. **B:** Only small changes in needle position can be accomplished once the tip is within deeper tissues. The direction of the needle tip that is within deeper tissues can be changed by grasping the needle shaft at the point where it enters the skin with one hand and at the needle hub with the other hand. By anchoring the shaft at the midpoint and moving the shaft in a direction opposite the direction the hub is moved, an arc is created along the shaft of the needle that can be directed toward the target (X).

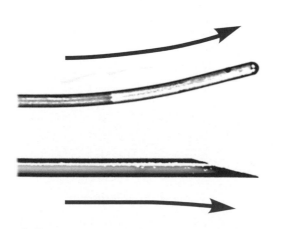

Figure 1-6.

Needle deviation during advancement. A straight, beveled-tip Quincke needle will veer slightly away from the bevel as it is advanced. A curved-tip needle will veer more dramatically toward the direction of the curved needle tip.

the needle to predictably deviate in the direction of the needle's tip and can be used to facilitate steering the needle toward the target (see Fig. 1-6). The size and shape of the curved needle tip differs from manufacturer to manufacturer, and only repeated use will familiarize the operator with the characteristics of each needle. A straight needle and precise coaxial technique are best in the majority of circumstances. However, when the actual target can not be aligned with the skin's surface using a coaxial technique, a curved needle can be quite helpful in steering the needle during advancement. This situation is often encountered during discography at the L5/S1 level. The plane of the intervertebral disc is angled in a cephalad-to-caudal direction and lies well below the pelvic brim. The sacral ala and iliac crest often lie directly in the path between the skin's surface and the posterolateral margin of the annulus fibrosis. A curved needle can be guided around the sacral ala and toward the disc behind this obstacle (see further description of lumbar discography in Chapter 9).

SUGGESTED READINGS

Ahn WS, Bahk JH, Lim YJ et al. The effect of introducer gauge, design and bevel direction on the deflection of spinal needles. *Anaesthesia.* 2002;57:1,007–1,011.

Baumgarten RK. Importance of the needle bevel during spinal and epidural anesthesia. *Reg Anesth.* 1995;20:234–238.

Drummond GB, Scott DH. The bevel and deflection of spinal needles. *Anesth Analg.* 1983;62:371.

Glazener EL. Deflection of spinal needles by the bevel. *Anaesthesia.* 1980;35:854–857.

Kapoor V, Rothfus WE, Grahovac SZ et al. Radicular pain avoidance during needle placement in lumbar diskography. *AJR Am J Roentgenol.* 2003;181:1,149–1,154.

Sitzman BT, Uncles DR. The effects of needle type, gauge, and tip bend on spinal needle deflection. *Anesth Analg.* 1996;82:297–301.

Stevens DS, Balatbat GR, Lee FM. Coaxial imaging technique for superior hypogastric plexus block. *Reg Anesth Pain Med.* 2000;25:643–647.

Radiation Safety

Overview

Pain practitioners have come to rely on fluoroscopy for image-guided injection for an increasing number of pain treatment techniques. Fluoroscopy employs ionizing radiation to produce the x-rays needed for imaging. Understanding the physics and biology underlying the biological effects of ionizing radiation is essential for pain practitioners to minimize radiation exposure during image-guided injection. The basic elements of the fluoroscopy unit are illustrated in Figure 2-1. X-rays emanate from an x-ray tube, typically positioned beneath the table and the patient to minimize radiation exposure. The x-rays pass through the table and the patient to strike the input phosphor of the image intensifier, where they are converted to visible light and in turn detected by an output phosphor that transfers the signal to a digital camera for visual display on a monitor or transfer to film. The size and shape of the x-ray beam can be adjusted after exiting the x-ray tube and before entering the patient, from side to side by an adjustable linear collimator or in a circular, concentric fashion by an iris collimator. The c-arm allows variation in the axis of the x-ray beam in numerous planes relative to the patient.

Basic Radiation Physics

Radiation is energy radiated or transmitted as rays, waves, or in the form of particles. X-rays are one portion of the spectrum of electromagnetic radiation. As x-rays pass through matter, they impart enough energy to dislodge electrons (ionizing radiation), yielding free radicals that can lead to harmful biological effects. In radiography, it is the x-rays that penetrate the body without effect that emerge to strike an image intensifier where they are converted to vis-

ible light and can be displayed on a monitor or transferred to film, producing an image based on x-ray penetrability of various tissues.

Several factors and definitions are central to any basic understanding of radiation safety. The biological effects of ionizing radiation are proportional to the time of exposure, whereas radiation exposure is inversely proportional to the *square* of the distance from the radiation source. Radiation exposure is expressed as roentgen or coulomb per kilogram, whereas the energy absorbed from radiation is expressed as radiation absorbed dose (rad) or as gray (Gy). Because different types of radiation can have different biological effects, units of exposure are converted from rad to radiation equivalent in man (rem) or Sievert (Sv). The units used to express radiation exposure are listed in Table 2-1. For x-rays, 1 roentgen (R) ~ 1 rad ~ 1 rem.

The electrical input to the tube that generates the x-rays can be varied to produce x-rays that differ in number and energy. Increased current applied to the x-ray tube (expressed as milliamps or mA) produces more x-rays, and the more x-rays that strike the image intensifier, the darker the image. Lengthening the exposure time will also increase the number of x-rays reaching the image intensifier, thus variations in current and exposure time are expressed as mAs (mA × seconds). Increased voltage (expressed as kilovoltage peak or kVp) applied to the x-ray tube results in x-ray emission at higher energy levels (i.e., with greater ability to penetrate). In general, high kVp (75 to 125 kVp) and low mA (50 to 1,200 mA) are employed for fluoroscopy with short exposure times. This combination optimizes image quality while minimizing radiation exposure. High kVp/low mA combinations expose the patient to significantly less radiation than low kVp/high mA combinations. Modern fluoroscopy units typically employ automatic brightness control (ABC), which automatically adjusts kVp and mA to yield optimal brightness and contrast.

The x-rays generated during fluoroscopy are a form of ionizing radiation and have the potential to produce significant biological effects. Small doses of ionizing radiation can produce molecular changes that take years to manifest in the form of cancerous transformation. Exposure to low doses of ionizing radiation is likely inconsequential because normal cellular mechanisms repair the damage. The International Committee on Radiation Safety Protection (ICRP) has produced estimates of the maximum permissible dose (MPD) of

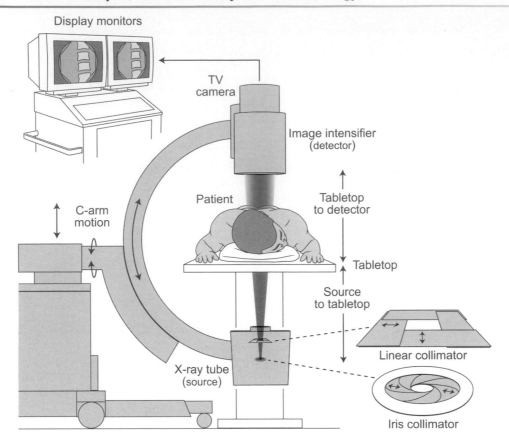

Figure 2-1.
Diagram of the components of a typical fluoroscopy unit.

annual radiation to various organs (Table 2-2). Exposure below these levels is unlikely to lead to any significant effects, but the ICRP recommends that workers should not receive more than 10% of the MPD.

Use of fluoroscopy for interventional procedures grew rapidly during the late 1980s, leading to increased concerns about radiation exposure. In 1994, the U.S. Food and Drug Administration (FDA) issued a public health advisory about serious radiation-related skin injuries resulting from some fluoroscopic procedures. Today's equipment and techniques have reduced the risks of radiation exposure dramatically. Radiation exposure during a typical epidural steroid injection carried out with fluoroscopy and assuming the practitioner is at least 1 m from the x-ray tube has been reported to be as low as 0.03 mR. In contrast, the typical entrance skin exposure during fluoroscopy ranges from 1 to 10 R per minute. A typical single chest radiograph leads to a skin entrance exposure of 15 mR. Thus, 1 minute of continuous fluoroscopy at 2 R per minute is equivalent to the exposure during 130 chest radiographs. Minimum target organ radiation doses that lead to pathologic effects are shown in Table 2-3. Radiation dermatitis still occurs in fluoroscopists with unknown long-term consequences.

Table 2–1			
Units Used to Express Radiation Exposure and Dose			
Term	**Traditional Units**	**SI Units**	**Conversion**
Exposure	Roentgen (R)	Coulomb/kg (C/kg)	$1 \text{ R} = 2.5 \times 10^{-4} \text{ C/kg}$
Radiation absorbed dose	rad	Gray (Gy)	100 rad = 1 Gy
Radiation equivalent in man	rem	Sievert (Sv)	100 rem = 1 Sv

Table 2–2
Annual Maximum Permissible Radiation Doses

Area/Organ	Annual Maximum Permissible Dose
Thyroid	50 rem (500 mSv)
Extremities	50 rem (500 mSv)
Lens of the eye	15 rem (150 mSv)
Gonads	50 rem (500 mSv)
Whole body	5 rem (50 mSv)
Pregnant women	0.5 rem to fetus (5 mSv)

Data from the National Council on Radiation Protection and Measurements (NCRP). Report No. 116. *Limitation of exposure to ionizing radiation.* Bethesda, MD: NCRP Publications; 1993.

Minimizing Patient Radiation Exposure

Minimize Dose and Time

Practitioners using ionizing radiation should adhere to the ALARA ("as low as reasonably achievable") principle, combining optimal technique and shielding to minimize patient and personnel exposure. Because no dose of ionizing radiation is without biological effects and can be considered absolutely safe, radiographs should be used only when necessary, and the dose and exposure time should be limited. Dose is a factor of both the number of x-rays (proportional to mA × seconds of exposure) and the energy of the x-rays (proportional to kVp). Modern fluoroscopy units employ ABC, which automatically controls mA and kVp settings to optimize brightness and contrast while minimizing dose. However, if you choose to use fluoroscopy in manual mode (e.g., to increase penetration in an obese patient), the kVp should be increased while minimizing mA. For an equivalent increase in exposure, the mA must be doubled, whereas the kVp must be raised only 15%. When using ABC mode, the only element under practitioner control is the exposure time, and this should be held to the minimum required to complete the procedure. Short pulses of exposure rather than continuous exposure should be employed whenever feasible. Continuous fluoroscopy in the form of movies (cineradiography) exposes patients to markedly higher doses than brief spot images. Many modern units include an option termed *pulse* mode for use in place of a continuous technique: This mode substitutes brief, periodic spot images separated by an interval without exposure (e.g., a new image is displayed one to two times per second). Use of this mode in place of continuous fluoroscopy can reduce overall exposure dramatically and is suitable for procedures in the pain clinic where continuous fluoroscopy is needed (e.g., while threading an epidural catheter or spinal cord stimulation lead).

Optimize the Position of the X-ray Tube

Radiation exposure to the patient is best minimized by ensuring optimal distance between patient and the x-ray tube (Fig. 2-2). When the x-ray tube is positioned close to the patient, a small area of skin will be exposed to radiation, but due to the close proximity of the x-rays, the dose that this smaller area will be exposed to is much higher. When the tube is positioned further from the patient, a larger area is exposed to a smaller dose of radiation. The x-ray tube should be positioned as far from the patient as possible, without including unnecessary structures in the field of view.

Employ Shielding Whenever Possible

The use of lead shielding can prevent exposure of regions adjacent to the area that is to be imaged from being exposed to any ionizing radiation. Small lead shields can be placed on the table underneath the patient, directly in front of the x-ray beam *before* it penetrates the patient to protect the gonads or the fetus, in the rare instance where fluoroscopy is necessary in a pregnant patient. Although lead shields should be readily available in the fluoroscopy suite, they are seldom practical for use during image-guided injection of the lumbosacral spine because the shield would lie directly in the path of the structures to be imaged.

Table 2–3
Minimum Target Organ Radiation Doses to Produce Organ Pathologic Effects

Organ	Dose (rad)	Dose (Gy)	Results
Eye lens	200	2	Cataract formation
Skin	500	5	Erythema
	700	7	Permanent alopecia
Whole body	200–700	2–7	Hematopoietic failure (4–6 wk)
	700–5,000	7–50	Gastrointestinal failure (3–4 d)
	5,000–10,000	50–100	Cerebral edema (1–2 d)

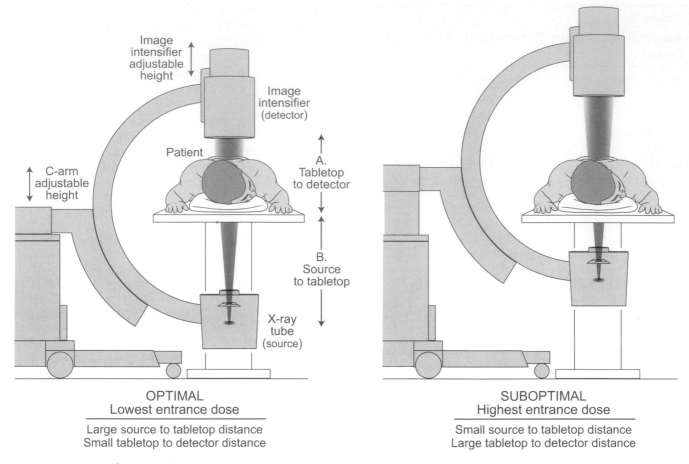

Figure 2-2.
Optimal spacing between the x-ray source and the patient to minimize radiation exposure.

Employ Collimation

Fluoroscopy units have built-in mechanisms that allow the emitted x-ray beam to be reduced in size and changed in shape (or *collimated*) so the area of the patient exposed is minimized. All units have both linear and circular collimation. Linear collimation employs shutters that can be moved in from either side of the exposure field and are helpful in imaging long, thin structures such as the spine (Fig. 2-3). Circular or "iris" collimation can be helpful when a small, circular area is to be imaged (Fig. 2-4). Collimation is also helpful in optimizing image quality because the ABC mode attempts to optimize the image quality by taking into account the exposure needed across the entire field of exposure; it is often difficult to visualize radiodense and radiolucent areas in the same image. Useful employment of collimation can exclude areas of greatly varying radiodensity to improve image quality by reducing the range of densities included in the field. Two good examples are imaging of the thoracic spine, where the large density differences between the spine and the adjacent air-filled lungs can make it difficult to see the bony elements of the spine with any resolution. Linear

collimation to limit the field to the spine itself will dramatically improve the image quality. Likewise, imaging in the cervical spine is fraught with the same difficulties when the air on either side of the neck is included in the x-ray field (see Fig. 2-3). Either linear collimation or circular collimation (see Fig. 2-4) can be used to limit the field to the area of interest, improving image quality and reducing radiation exposure. Modern fluoro units may also allow for *magnification* of the image by electronically magnifying the area of interest. Magnification allows better visualization of a smaller area, but leads to increased radiation exposure as the system increases output to compensate for losses in gain. To minimize the dose to the patient, the largest field of view, in conjunction with the tightest collimation should be employed.

Minimizing Practitioner Exposure

Employ Proper Shielding

Only the personnel needed to conduct the procedure should be in the fluoroscopy suite. All personnel should be

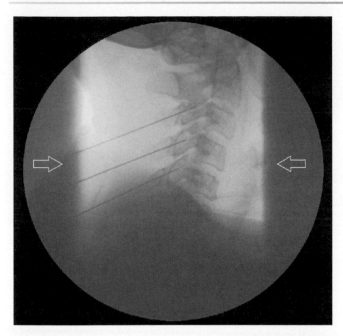

Figure 2-3.
Use of adjustable (linear) collimator to decrease radiation exposure to the patient, while improving image resolution by decreasing the range of tissue density included in the image field.

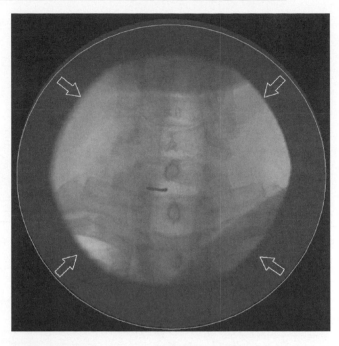

Figure 2-4.
Use of adjustable (iris) collimator to limit the field to the area of interest reduces radiation exposure to the patient and improves image resolution by decreasing the range of tissue density included in the image field.

shielded with lead aprons *before* use of fluoroscopy begins. The practitioner using the fluoroscopy unit should alert everyone in the room that he or she is about to begin and ensure that personnel are shielded. Routine use of thyroid shields can minimize the long-term risk of thyroid cancer. Although protective lead gloves can reduce the exposure of the hands to radiation, they can produce a false sense of security. When leaded gloves are employed and the practitioner's hands are in the field of exposure, units with ABC will increase their output to compensate for the radiodense leaded gloves, and negate their protective effects. Using techniques that eliminate the practitioner's hands from direct exposure within the x-ray field should be used at all times. Protective eyeglasses are available that dramatically reduce eye exposure during fluoroscopy; leaded eyewear is recommended for practitioners who accumulate monthly readings on collar badges above 400 mrem (4 Sv). Levels of exposure in this range are typically encountered only in areas where continuous cine-angiography is conducted frequently (e.g., the cardiac catheterization laboratory).

Practitioner Position

The practitioner must understand the geometry of the radiation path as it passes from the x-ray tube to the image intensifier and adopt positions that minimize their exposure during fluoroscopy (Fig. 2-5). The dose drops proportion-

ally to the square of the distance from the x-ray source. Thus, standing as far from the x-ray tube as practical is the first means to minimize exposure. Using an intravenous extension tube and taking a step back from the table during periods where contrast is injected under continuous or live fluoroscopy will reduce exposure. When the x-ray tube is rotated to obtain a lateral image, the practitioner should step completely away from the table beneath the x-ray tube and out of the path of the x-ray beam or move to the side of the table of the image intensifier. Inverting the c-arm so the x-ray tube is above the table and the image intensifier is below the table is a means used by some practitioners to increase the c-arm's range of lateral movement beyond the typical 45 to 55 degrees allowed by the unit. This practice dramatically increases exposure to both patient and practitioner by bringing them in close proximity to the x-ray source.

Optimizing Image Quality

Modern fluoroscopy units use ABC, which automatically adjusts mA and kVp to optimize image brightness and contrast while minimizing radiation exposure. These controls can be adjusted separately. Increased kVp produces x-rays of higher energy that penetrate without attenuation, thus the resulting image is brighter with less contrast between different tissues, thereby reducing image detail. The clarity of small structures, or image detail, can be improved by

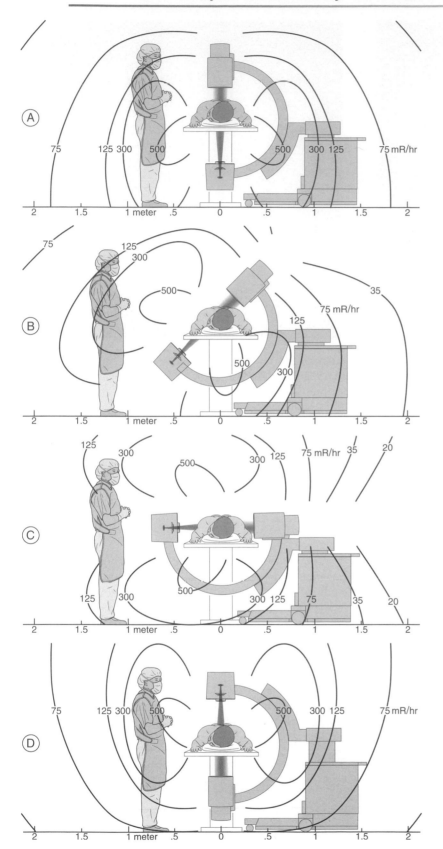

Figure 2-5.
Radiation exposure dosage during fluoroscopy. **A:** During routine use in the anterior-posterior plane, the x-ray tube (source) should be positioned below the patient and the detector above the patient to minimize radiation exposure to both the patient and the practitioner. **B:** The oblique projection results in markedly increased exposure to the practitioner. **C:** During use in the lateral projection, the practitioner should step completely behind the x-ray tube (source) to minimize radiation exposure. When it is necessary to work close to the patient during lateral fluoroscopy, the practitioner should move to the side of the table opposite the x-ray tube to minimize exposure. **D:** Radiation exposure to both patient and practitioner is dramatically increased when the x-ray tube (source) is inverted above the patient. Some practitioners invert the c-arm to allow for more extreme lateral angle (e.g., rotation beyond 35 to 45 degrees oblique to the side opposite the c-arm is not possible without inverting the c-arm on some units). Radiation exposure can be reduced by rotating the patient on the table and keeping the x-ray source below the table. (Adapted with the assistance of Philips Medical Systems USA, Seattle, WA, based on radiation exposure data for the Pulsera 9-inch mobile c-arm.)

lowering kVP, reducing the distance between the patient and the image intensifier, and by using collimation to limit the field of exposure to only those structures of interest. Fluoroscopic images also have less sharpness at the periphery of the image due to a falloff in brightness and spatial resolution, a phenomenon called *vignetting*. Placing the structure of interest in the center of the image will yield maximum image detail. Finally, *pincushion distortion* occurs toward the periphery of the image because the x-rays emanate from a spherical surface and are detected on a flat surface. This results in an effect much like a fisheye camera lens with a splaying outward of objects toward the periphery of the image. This can lead to particular difficulties when attempting to advance a needle using a coaxial technique if the needle is toward the periphery of the image.

SUGGESTED READINGS

Berlin L. Malpractice issues in radiology: radiation-induced skin injuries and fluoroscopy. *AJR Am J Roentgenol.* 2001;178:153–157.

Fishman SM, Smith H, Meleger A et al. Radiation safety in pain medicine. *Reg Anesth Pain Med.* 2002;27:296–305.

Norris TG. Radiation safety in fluoroscopy. *Radiol Technol.* 2002;73:511–533.

U.S. Food and Drug Administration. *Public Health Advisory: Avoidance of Serious X-ray Induced Skin Injuries to Patients During Fluoroscopically-guided Procedures.* Rockville, MD: U.S. Food and Drug Administration, Center for Devices and Radiological Health; September 1994.

Radiographic Contrast Agents

Overview

Iodine is the only element that has proven satisfactory as an intravascular radiographic contrast medium (RCM). Iodine produces the radiopacity, whereas the other portions of the molecule act as the carriers for the iodine, improving solubility and reducing the toxicity of the final compound. Organic carriers of iodine are likely to remain in widespread use for the foreseeable future. During image-guided injection, injection of RCM can prove invaluable in determining the final location and distribution of the injectate (Figs. 3-1 to 3-3). Use of RCM can improve the safety of many techniques by allowing for detection of intravascular (Figs. 3-4 and 3-5), subdural (see Fig. 3-2), or intrathecal (see Fig. 3-3) needle location *before* local anesthetic or steroid are placed.

Pharmacology

Currently, there are four chemical varieties of iodinated RCM in widespread use: ionic monomers, nonionic monomers, ionic dimers, and nonionic dimers. On intravascular injection, all four are redistributed rapidly via capillary permeability to the extravascular space, they do not enter the interior of blood or tissue cells, and they are rapidly excreted, more than 90% eliminated via glomerular filtration within 12 hours of administration. None of the four varieties have marked pharmacologic actions. All RCM agents come in a range of concentrations that vary according to the radiopacity. Because iodine is the element that is responsible for the radiopacity, the iodine concentration in milligrams per milliliter represents the radiopacity. The nonionic monomers are now used almost exclusively in pain medicine; the nonionic dimers offer increased radiopacity at low osmolar concentrations, but are not yet in widespread clinical use.

There are several important chemical properties that determine the characteristics of RCM in clinical use. *Osmolality* depends on the number of particles of solute in solution and is highest for the ionic contrast agents. Adverse reactions, particularly discomfort on injection, have been reduced dramatically with the advent of low-osmolar RCM. Contrast media with osmolality below 500 mosm per kg of water are virtually painless. *Radiopacity* depends on the iodine concentration of the solution, and therefore, on the number of iodine atoms per molecule and the concentration of the iodine-carrying molecule in solution. Digital subtraction electronically enhances the image, reducing the amount of contrast medium needed by a factor of twofold to threefold. With use of digital subtraction, RCM with as little as 150 to 200 mg per mL of iodine can be used even for intra-arterial use. Ionic molecules dissociate into cation and anion in solution. Nonionicity, or a molecule that does not dissociate in solution, is essential for myelography or use along the neuraxis, where placement within the CSF is possible during injection. The chemical properties of two of the most common RCM used in clinical practice are compared in Table 3-1.

The most frequently used ionic monomers are diatrizoate (Urografin), iothalamate (Conray), and metrizoate (Isopaque). All ionic monomers are the salts of meglumine or sodium as the cation and a radiopaque tri-iodinated fully substituted benzene ring as the anion. The ionic monomers are still used for intravenous pyelography and similar applications; however, they have been completely replaced by the low-osmolar, nonionic RCM for many applications, including intrathecal administration. The most common nonionic monomers in clinical use include iohexol (Omnipaque), iopamidol (Niopam), and ioversol (Optiray). The nonionic monomers appeared in the 1970s, and now represent the most common RCM in clinical use. They are more stable in solution and less toxic than the ionic monomers.

Adverse Reactions to Radiographic Contrast Media

Modern contrast agents have reduced, but not eliminated, the risk of adverse reactions. To minimize the risk, RCM should be used in the smallest concentrations and in the smallest total dose that will allow adequate visualization. Adverse reactions associated with RCM can be divided

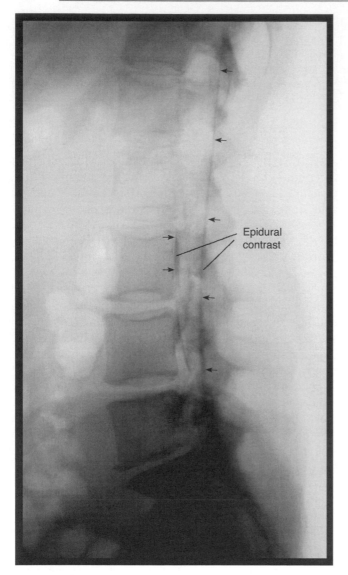

Figure 3-1.
Epidural contrast injection. This typical lateral lumbar epiduro-gram demonstrates the "double-line" or "railroad track" appearance of radiographic contrast in the anterior and posterior epidural space (*arrows*). (Reprinted from Rathmell JP, Torian D, Song T. Lumbar epidurography. *Reg Anesth Pain Med.* 2000;25:541, with permission.)

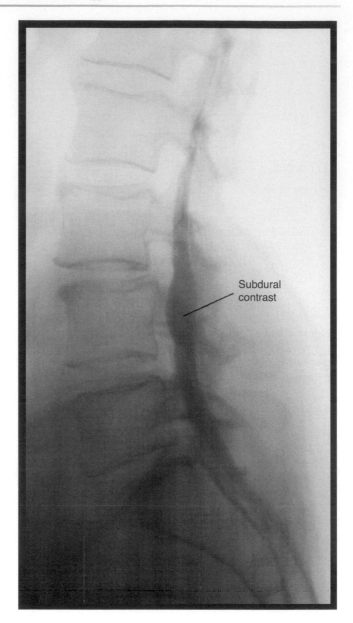

Figure 3-2.
Subdural contrast injection. Injection of contrast in the subdural (epiarachnoid) space is recognized by the loculated appearance of the contrast collection on this lateral radiograph of the lumbar spine. Although the contrast does not extend to the anterior portion of the thecal sac, it is not limited to the epidural space. (Reprinted from Ajar A, Rathmell JP, Mukerji S. The subdural compartment. *Reg Anesth Pain Med.* 2002;27:73, with permission.)

into idiosyncratic anaphylactoid reactions, nonidiosyncratic reactions, and combined reactions. The risk of adverse reactions is significantly greater with use of high-osmolar, ionic agents when compared with low-osmolar, nonionic agents. This discussion is limited to the risks associated with low-osmolar, nonionic agents because they are used almost exclusively in pain medicine applications.

Idiosyncratic Anaphylactoid Reactions

Idiosyncratic reactions are the most feared, as well as the most serious and even fatal, complications associated with

RCM. At present, we cannot predict or prevent this type of reaction reliably, and they occur without warning. These reactions usually begin within 5 minutes of injection, and may be mild and self-limited or proceed rapidly to life-threatening cardiovascular collapse. The risk of anaphylactoid reaction is increased in patients with previous reaction to RCM (sixfold), in asthmatics (eightfold), in allergic and atopic patients (fourfold), and in those with advanced heart disease (threefold) (Table 3-2).

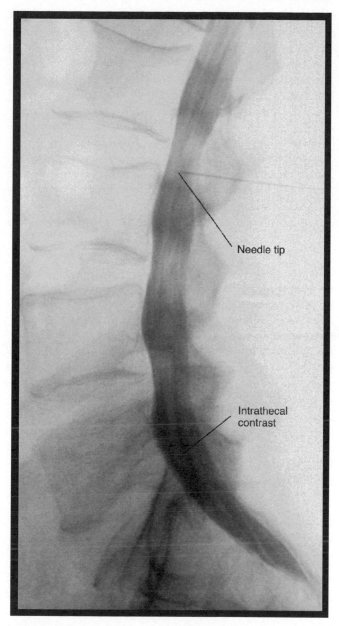

Figure 3-3.
Intrathecal contrast injection. This typical myelogram demonstrates contrast within the thecal sac on this lateral radiograph of the lumbar spine. The spinal cord and exiting nerve roots are visible as hypodense regions within the contrast collection. (Reprinted from Rathmell JP, Torian D, Song T. Lumbar epidurography. *Reg Anesth Pain Med.* 2000;25:543, with permission.)

Nonidiosyncratic Anaphylactoid Reactions

Nonidiosyncratic reactions can be divided into chemotoxic reactions, those due to chemical reactions to the iodine-carrying molecule, and osmotoxic reactions, or those caused by high osmolality of the contrast medium. These nonidiosyncratic reactions are dose dependent; therefore, this type of reaction should be exceedingly rare in patients receiving the small volumes of RCM required to facilitate needle localization during image-guided pain treatment.

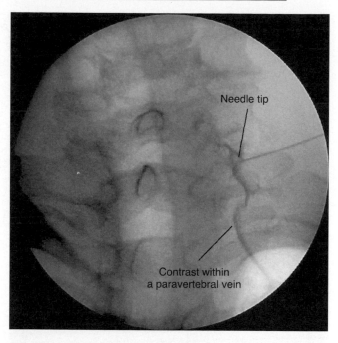

Figure 3-4.
Intravenous contrast injection. Intravenous contrast injection is typically not seen on still images because the contrast material is rapidly diluted in the bloodstream. During real-time or live fluoroscopy, intravenous contrast injection appears as in this anterior-posterior radiograph of the cervical spine taken during cervical transforaminal injection. The contrast can be seen flowing toward the heart with the venous blood.

Chemotoxic reactions are rare and may result in direct organ toxicity and include cardiac (direct and prolonged decrease in cardiac contractility), neurologic (seizures), and renal toxicity (oliguria, impaired creatinine clearance, and reduced glomerular filtration rate that may progress to acute renal failure).

Osmotoxic reactions were much more common with the high-osmolar contrast media, where the osmolality of the RCM can reach several times that of physiologic osmolality of 300 mosm per kg H_2O (see Table 3-1). Osmotoxic reactions have been dramatically reduced with the advent of low-osmolar, nonionic agents such as iohexol and should be exceedingly rare after administration of the small volumes used in pain medicine applications. Hyperosmolar reactions include erythrocyte damage (hemolysis), endothelial damage (capillary leak and edema), vasodilation (flushing, warmth, hypotension, cardiovascular collapse), hypervolemia, and direct cardiac depression (reduced cardiac contractility). The relative incidence of various adverse reactions to RCM is listed in Table 3-3.

Recognition and Treatment of Reactions to Radiographic Contrast Media

Reactions can be generally grouped as mild, moderate, or severe. The incidence of these reactions following the

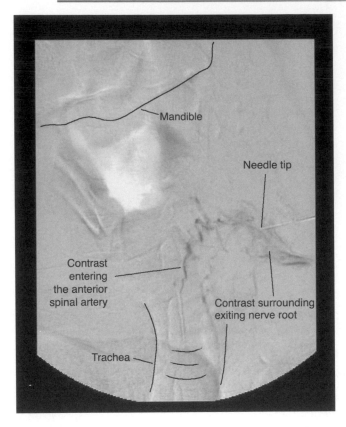

Figure 3-5.
Intra-arterial contrast injection (digital subtraction). Intra-arterial contrast injection is typically not seen on still images because the contrast material is rapidly diluted in the bloodstream. During real-time or live fluoroscopy, intravenous contrast injection appears as in this anterior-posterior digital subtraction radiograph of the cervical spine taken during cervical transforaminal injection. The contrast can be seen flowing away from the heart toward the end organ (in this image, toward the spinal cord) with the arterial blood. Use of digital subtraction cine-radiography allows for detection of intravascular injection with small doses of radiographic contrast material. (Adapted from Rathmell JP, Aprill C, Bogduk N. Cervical transforaminal injection of steroids. *Anesthesiology.* 2004;100:1,597, with permission.)

small volumes of RCM used in pain medicine has not been detailed, but the incidence following intravenous administration of larger volumes of contrast is given here. Mild reactions occur in 5% to 15% of those receiving intravenous contrast, and include flushing anxiety, nausea, arm pain, pruritus, vomiting, headache, and mild urticaria. These are generally mild and self-limiting, and require no specific treatment. Occasionally, an oral antihistamine (diphenhydramine 25 mg) can be useful in managing pruritus and anxiety. More serious reactions occur in 0.5% to 2% of those receiving intravenous contrast and include more pronounced severity of mild symptoms, as well as moderate degrees of hypotension and bronchospasm. Suggested treatments for moderate reactions are given in Table 3-4.

Severe reactions are life threatening; occur in less than 0.04% of those receiving intravenous RCM; and include convulsions, unconsciousness, laryngeal edema, severe bronchospasm, pulmonary edema, severe cardiac arrhythmias, and cardiovascular collapse. Treatment of these life-threatening reactions is urgent, necessitating the immediate availability of full resuscitation equipment and trained personnel, along with a practiced routine for responding to these rare events. The airway must be secured, and oxygen, mechanical ventilation, external cardiac massage, and electrical cardiac defibrillation must be administered as required. Death may ensue following this type of severe adverse reaction; the incidence is not known with accuracy, but likely lies between 1/14,000 to 1/170,000 intravenous administrations of RCM.

Prevention of Reactions to Radiographic Contrast Media

Recognition of the factors that predispose patients to adverse reactions when receiving RCM is the first step in prevention (see Table 3-2). The risk of reaction is increased

Table 3–1
Comparison of Two Common Radiographic Contrast Agents Used in Clinical Practice[a]

Chemical Composition	Trade Name	Iodine (mg/mL)	Osmolality (mosm/kg H_2O)	Viscosity (cps @ 37°C)	RCM Agent Type
Sodium/meglumine diatrizoate	Urografin 150	146	710	1.4	Ionic, high-osmolar
Sodium/meglumine diatrizoate	Urografin 325	325	1,650	3.3	Ionic, high-osmolar
Iohexol	Omnipaque 180	180	360	2.0	Nonionic, low-osmolar
Iohexol	Omnipaque 300	300	640	6.1	Nonionic, low-osmolar

RCM, radiographic contrast media.
[a] The ionic, high-osmolar agent diatrizoate and the nonionic, low-osmolar, agent iohexol. Iohexol (180 mg/mL) is the agent used almost exclusively in pain medicine applications. This agent provides a nonionic, low-osmolar RCM that balances a low risk of adverse reaction, safety for intrathecal administration, and sufficient radio-opacity for identifying intravascular and intrathecal placement.

Table 3–2

Incidence of Severe Adverse Drug Reactions

Clinical History	Severe ADR (%)[a]
No history of allergy or previous ADR to RCM	0.03
Renal disease	0.04
Diabetes mellitus	0.05
Heart disease	0.10
History of allergy	0.10
Atopy	0.11
History of previous ADR to RCM	0.18
Asthma	0.23

ADR, adverse drug reaction; RCM, radiographic contrast media.
[a]ADR following intravenous injection of low-osmolar, nonionic RCM.
Katayama H, Yamaguchi K, Kozuka T et al. Adverse reactions to ionic and non-ionic contrast media. A report from the Japanese Committee on the Safety of Contrast Media. *Radiology.* 1990;175:621–628.

in those with previous reaction to RCM (sixfold), in asthmatics (eightfold), in allergic and atopic patients (fourfold), and in patients with advanced heart disease (threefold). If there is any chance that the injectate will end up in the subarachnoid space, then a low-osmolar, nonionic contrast agent must be used. Infrequent deaths have been reported following the inadvertent intrathecal administration of

Table 3–3

Type and Relative Incidence of Adverse Drug Reactions

Patient characteristics in trial	
Total number of patients	163,363
Total ADRs	3.13%
Total severe ADRs	0.04%
Death	(1)

Symptoms	% of ADR[a]
Nausea	1.04
Heat	0.92
Vomiting	0.45
Urticaria	0.47
Flushing	0.16
Venous pain	0.05
Coughing	0.15
Dyspnea	0.04

ADR, adverse drug reaction
[a]ADR following intravenous injection of low-osmolar, nonionic radiographic contrast media.
Adapted from Katayama H, Yamaguchi K, Kozuka T et al. Adverse reactions to ionic and non-ionic contrast media. A report from the Japanese Committee on the Safety of Contrast Media. *Radiology.* 1990;175:621–628, with permission.

ionic RCM. Most pain medicine practitioners have adopted the universal use of a low-osmolar, nonionic RCM in a moderate concentration (e.g., iohexol 180 mg per mL) for all applications.

There is no known premedication regimen that can reliably eliminate the risk of severe reactions to RCM. The most common strategies suggested combine pretreatment with corticosteroids (e.g., oral prednisone 50-mg doses 12 and 2 hours before RCM administration) and antihistamines (e.g., oral diphenhydramine 50-mg doses 1 to 2 hours before RCM administration). Some authors recommend addition of H_2-antagonists (e.g., oral ranitidine). This approach has proven to reduce the incidence of subsequent adverse reactions in those with a history of previous reaction to high-osmolar contrast agents; however, it is less clear whether prophylactic treatment is needed prior to use of a low-osmolar, nonionic contrast agents such as iohexol. Patients believed to be at greater than usual risk are listed in Table 3-5. It has been our practice to avoid radiographic contrast altogether in those at elevated risk for adverse reaction. Most procedures in pain medicine can be carried out safely without use of radiographic contrast. In some instances (e.g., epidural placement), the location can be established using loss of resistance alone, and final needle position can be verified using anterior-posterior and lateral radiography without contrast. However, some injections should not be attempted without radiographic contrast injection (e.g., transforaminal injection); in this case, injection of contrast under live or real-time fluoroscopy (with or without digital subtraction) is the only means to detect intra-arterial needle location (see Fig. 3-5) and to prevent catastrophic injection of particulate steroid directly into critical vessels supplying the spinal cord. Performing interlaminar epidural steroid injection without contrast may well be a safe and effective alternative to transforaminal injection in the patient with greater than usual risk for adverse reaction to RCM.

Table 3–4

Suggested Treatment for Reactions to Radiographic Contrast Media of Moderate Severity

Adverse Reaction	Suggested Treatment
Urticaria	Diphenhydramine 25–50 mg PO, IM, or IV
Anxiety	Diazepam 5–10 mg PO or midazolam 1–2 mg IV
Bronchospasm	Mild: Inhaled albuterol Severe: Hydrocortisone 100 mg IV Epinephrine 0.05–0.1 mg SQ, IM, IV

Table 3–5

Patients Considered at Greater than Usual Risk of Severe Adverse Reactions to Radiographic Contrast Media

Those with a history of previous adverse reactions to RCM (excluding mild flushing and nausea)

Asthmatics

Allergic and atopic patients

Cardiac patients with congestive heart failure, unstable arrhythmia, or recent myocardial infarction

Patients with diabetic nephropathy or renal failure of any etiology

Feeble, elderly patients

Those with severe, general debility or dehydration

Extremely anxious patients

Patients with specific hematologic or metabolic disorders (e.g., sickle cell anemia, polycythemia, multiple myeloma, pheochromocytoma)

RCM, radiographic contrast media.
Adapted from Grainger RG. Intravascular radiologic iodinated contrast media. In: Grainger RG, Allison DJ, Adam A et al., eds. *Grainger & Allison's Diagnostic Radiology.* 4th ed. New York: Churchill Livingstone; 2001, with permission.

SUGGESTED READINGS

Ajar A, Rathmell JP, Mukerji S. The subdural compartment. *Reg Anesth Pain Med.* 2002;27:72–76.

American College of Radiology. *Manual on Contrast Media.* 4th ed. Reston, VA: American College of Radiology; 1999.

Dawson P, Cosgrove DO, Grainger RG, eds. *Textbook of Contrast Media.* Oxford, England: ISIS Medical Media; 1999.

Grainger RG. Intravascular radiologic iodinated contrast media. In: Grainger RG, Allison DJ, Adam A et al., eds. *Grainger & Allison's Diagnostic Radiology.* 4th ed. New York: Churchill Livingstone; 2001.

Greenberger PA, Patterson R. The prevention of immediate generalized reactions to radiocontrast media in high-risk patients. *Clin Immunol.* 1991,87:867–872.

Katayama H, Yamaguchi K, Kozuka T et al. Adverse reactions to ionic and non-ionic contrast media. A report from the Japanese Committee on the Safety of Contrast Media. *Radiology.* 1990;175:621–628.

Rathmell JP, Torian D, Song T. Lumbar epidurography. *Reg Anesth Pain Med.* 2000;25:540–545.

Spring DB, Bettman MA, Barkan HE. Deaths related to iodinated contrast media reported spontaneously to U.S. Food and Drug Administration 1978–1994: effect of availability of low osmolality contrast media. *Radiology.* 1997;204:333–337.

Thomsen HS, Muller RN, Mattrey RF, eds. *Trends in Contrast Media.* Berlin: Springer-Verlag; 1999.

CHAPTER 4

Pharmacology of Agents Used During Image-Guided Injection

Overview

The most common agents used during image-guided injection in the pain clinic are local anesthetics and adrenocortical steroids (glucocorticoids). Most injection techniques used in pain medicine are aimed at depositing a potent steroidal anti-inflammatory drug adjacent to a region where there is presumed to be inflammation causing pain. Local anesthetics are a core part of the armamentarium for anesthetizing the needle track during placement and producing neural blockade. In certain circumstances (e.g., neurolytic celiac plexus block for pain associated with intra-abdominal malignancy), neurolytic solutions are used to effect long-lasting or "permanent" neural blockade. In this section, we discuss the pharmacology of these drugs.

Pharmacology of Local Anesthetics

Mechanism of Action

Local anesthetics completely abolish neuronal signal transmission by binding reversibly within the sodium channel on neuronal membranes. They produce dense sensory blockade in the region injected when infiltrated into the skin and subcutaneous tissues, or within the territory of the specific nerve when injected around a major peripheral nerve. When local anesthetics are injected along the neuraxis, they produce segmental anesthesia in a dermatomal distribution when placed in the epidural space, and profound sensory and motor block of the trunk and lower extremities when placed within the thecal sac.

Local Anesthetic Structure and Function

Local anesthetics have three basic building blocks: a lipophilic aromatic end (benzene ring), a hydrophilic tertiary amine end, and an intermediate chain connecting the two ends. The chemical connection between the intermediate chain and the aromatic end allows us to classify local anesthetics as either "esters" or "amides." Figure 4-1 illustrates these basic chemical building blocks. Amino amides are chemically more stable and have less potential for allergic reactions than the esters. The properties of amide and ester local anesthetics are compared in Table 4-1. The two most common agents used for image-guided injection are the amide local anesthetics lidocaine and bupivacaine. The onset and duration of the common local anesthetics are illustrated in Figure 4-2.

Local Anesthetic Dose Versus Site of Injection

The doses and expected distribution of neural blockade of local anesthetics are second nature to the anesthesiologist; those with less familiarity with use of local anesthetics must gain some familiarity with their use and potential toxicities before attempting to use these drugs during image-guided injection. The typical doses of lidocaine and bupivacaine used to produce local anesthesia, peripheral nerve block, and epidural or spinal anesthesia are compared in Table 4-2.

Local Anesthetic Allergy

Local anesthetics have low allergic potential. The majority of "allergic reactions" reported by patients are misinterpretations of the cause of symptoms following local anesthetic injection. A frequent scenario reported by a patient as "an allergy to local anesthetic" occurs when they have received a local anesthetic injection in a dental office. On close questioning, the symptoms are usually attributable to intravascular injection of local anesthetic containing epinephrine as a vasoconstrictor (e.g., racing of the heart, palpitations, even a feeling of doom). Rarely are actual allergic manifestations (e.g., urticaria, bronchospasm, anaphylaxis) part of the history.

Local Anesthetic Toxicity

Local anesthetics are associated with life-threatening toxicities. As serum levels of local anesthetic rise, symptoms of excitation of the central nervous system appear, first in the form of tinnitus and dizziness followed by generalized seizures (Fig. 4-3). At higher serum levels, local anesthetics produce cardiac arrhythmias and cardiovascular collapse.

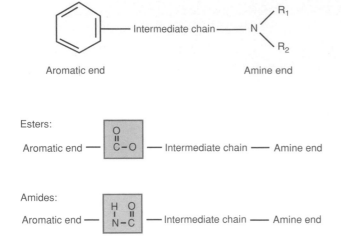

Figure 4-1.
Structure of the local anesthetic molecule. (Adapted from Viscomi CM. Pharmacology of local anesthetics. In: Rathmell JP, Neal JM, Viscomi CV, eds. *Requisites in Anesthesiology: Regional Anesthesia.* Philadelphia: Elsevier Health Sciences; 2004:14, with permission.)

Recommended maximal doses of local anesthetics are shown in Table 4-3.

It is important to keep in mind that even small doses of local anesthetic can have profound effects when injected in specific locations: Intrathecal injection of 150 mg of lidocaine or 20 mg of bupivacaine may well lead to total spinal anesthesia and the need for ventilatory support until the anesthetic level recedes. Likewise, direct intra-arterial injection of even a few milligrams of local anesthetic into the vertebral artery can cause immediate generalized seizures because the local anesthetic travels directly to the brain in high concentration. Any practitioner performing injection techniques with local anesthetics must be familiar with these toxicities and their management, and work in a facility equipped to handle such adverse events.

Pharmacology of Steroid Preparations

The pharmacology of the corticosteroids is complex, and this group of drugs affects almost all body systems. In phar-macologic doses (e.g., exceeding the rate of endogenous steroid production of approximately 20 mg per day of hydrocortisone or the equivalent), glucocorticoids decrease inflammation by stabilizing leukocyte lysosomal membranes; preventing release of destructive acid hydrolases from leukocytes; inhibiting macrophage accumulation in inflamed areas; reducing leukocyte adhesion to capillary endothelium; reducing capillary wall permeability and edema formation; decreasing complement components; antagonizing histamine activity and release of kinins from substrates; and reducing fibroblast proliferation, collagen deposition, and subsequent scar tissue formation. Several long-acting steroid preparations are available for parenteral use in formulations approved for intramuscular administration. These parenteral formulations are widely used in image-guided injections for perineural and epidural administration, but none of the available formulations has been approved by any regulatory agency in the United States or internationally for these applications.

There are several available steroid preparations with prolonged duration of action. They are commercially available in solutions that are designed to be equipotent (i.e., a single milliliter of each commercially available solution should produce similar glucocorticoid effects). The equipotent doses for commonly used steroids are shown in Table 4-4.

Equivalent doses are approximations and may not apply to routes of administration other than the oral route. The duration of anti-inflammatory activity of glucocorticoids is approximately equal to the duration of suppression of the hypothalamic-pituitary-adrenal (HPA) axis. The duration of suppression of the HPA axis following intramuscular injection of steroid preparations commonly used for epidural injection is shown in Table 4-5.

All of the available long-acting glucocorticoid formulations contain a number of preservatives and excipients (benzyl alcohol, benzalkonium chloride, and edetate sodium are common in these solutions). The safety of subarachnoid administration of the steroids themselves, as well as their preservatives and excipients, has been questioned. The manufacturer of Depo-Medrol states that this preparation of methylprednisolone acetate should not be administered intrathecally due to association with "severe medical events" when administered by this route (arachnoiditis has been reported). Other adverse events associated with

Table 4–1		
Properties of Amide and Ester Local Anesthetic Agents		
	Esters	Amides
Metabolism	Plasma cholinesterase	Hepatic
Serum half-life	Shorter	Longer
Allergic potential	Low	Very low
Specific drugs	Procaine, chloroprocaine, cocaine, tetracaine	Lidocaine, mepivacaine, bupivacaine, ropivacaine, etodocaine, prilocaine

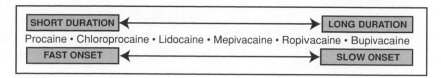

Figure 4-2.
Onset and duration of local anesthetics. (Adapted from Viscomi CM. Pharmacology of local anesthetics. In: Rathmell JP, Neal JM, Viscomi CV, eds. *Requisites in Anesthesiology: Regional Anesthesia*. Philadelphia: Elsevier Health Sciences; 2004:17, with permission.)

glucocorticoid administration are shown in Table 4-6. The vast majority of these adverse reactions are associated with long-term glucocorticoid administration. The most common adverse reactions after single-dose or short-course epidural administration of glucocorticoids include asymptomatic peripheral edema and increased insulin requirements in diabetic patients. All steroid preparations in use have some degree of mineralocorticoid effect, and the resultant fluid retention can lead to exacerbation of congestive heart failure (CHF) in those with chronic CHF. Finally, anaphylactoid reactions following glucocorticoid administration are rare but have been well described.

Much rhetoric has surrounded the use of particulate steroid preparations during transforaminal injection. Some practitioners have touted the use of betamethasone or triamcinolone over methylprednisolone acetate, citing the belief that the size of the particles is larger in the latter preparation. In the event the steroid was administered into a critical reinforcing artery supplying the spinal cord, theoretically the smaller particles could be less likely to cause spinal cord infarction. All available parenteral suspensions contain a wide and overlapping range of particle sizes; practitioners should not rely on the choice of steroid to eliminate the risk of direct intra-arterial injection.

Pharmacology of Neurolytic Solutions

The idea that chemical destruction of neural pathways can produce long-lasting pain relief has been around for many years. However, neurolytic blockade has met with limited success in treating most chronic pain conditions. Likely, the anatomic and functional changes that occur within the dorsal horn of the spinal cord and at higher centers within the brain lead to ongoing perception of pain even after destruction of the peripheral nerves that originally carried the nociceptive signals. Nonetheless, there are a number of neurolytic blocks that have proven beneficial and are still routinely performed. Foremost among efficacious neurolytic blocks is neurolytic celiac plexus block for the treatment of pain associated with intra-abdominal malignancy. Here, we briefly discuss the pharmacology of the two most common neurolytic agents: phenol and absolute alcohol.

Phenol

Phenol is the combination of carbolic acid, phenic acid, phenylic acid, phenyl hydroxide, hydroxybenzene, and oxybenzene. There is no commercially available phenol preparation, but a solution can be prepared by a compounding

Table 4–2

Typical Local Anesthetic Doses Used to Produce Neural Blockade[a]

Type of Block	Typical Drug Dose	
	Lidocaine	Bupivacaine
Local anesthesia (e.g., a 2-3 cm diameter area of skin)	10–40 mg (1–2 mL of 1%–2% solution)	2.5–10 mg (1–2 mL of 0.25%–0.50% solution)
Peripheral nerve block (e.g., lumbar selective nerve root block)	20–40 mg (1–2 mL of 2% solution)	5–10 mg (1–2 mL of 0.5% solution)
Epidural anesthesia (e.g., dense anesthesia for surgery on the lower extremity)	300–600 mg (20–30 mL of 1.5%–2% solution)	100–150 mg (20–30 mL of 0.5% solution)
Spinal anesthesia (e.g., dense anesthesia for surgery on the lower extremity)	50–100 mg (1–2 mL of 5% solution)	10–15 mg (1–2 mL of 0.825% solution)

[a]The drug doses shown are meant to illustrate the dramatic differences in drug dose required, depending on where the local anesthetic is placed. Even small doses of local anesthetic placed within the thecal sac (spinal anesthesia) can produce profound sensory and motor block that extends to the upper torso and, at higher doses, to the head and neck (total spinal anesthesia).

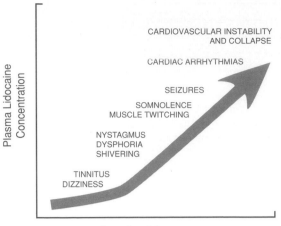

Figure 4-3.
Patient symptoms with progressive rise in plasma lidocaine levels. This symptom progression—from dizziness and tinnitus to generalized seizures followed by cardiovascular collapse at the highest plasma concentrations—occurs reliably with lidocaine. However, cardiovascular instability and collapse may present with the appearance of other signs or symptoms following intravascular injection of the more potent amide local anesthetic bupivacaine. (Adapted from Viscomi CM. Pharmacology of local anesthetics. In: Rathmell JP, Neal JM, Viscomi CV, eds. *Requisites in Anesthesiology: Regional Anesthesia.* Philadelphia: Elsevier Health Sciences; 2004:22, with permission.)

pharmacist from anhydrous phenol crystals available from chemical supply houses. The limit of solubility of phenol in water is approximately 6.67%. Phenol is highly soluble in glycerin and in radiographic contrast solutions. We have tested the stability of 12% phenol in iohexol 180 mg per mL and found that no precipitation or release of free iodine occurs over 30 days at room temperature. We prefer mixing phenol in radiographic contrast so that the pattern of spread of the neurolytic solution can be monitored radiographically throughout the injection. Solutions of aqueous phenol, phenol in glycerin, and phenol in iohexol are all markedly vis-

Table 4–3	
Recommended Maximum Local Anesthetic Doses[a]	
Anesthetic	**Maximum Recommended Dose**
Lidocaine	4–5 mg/kg
Mepivacaine	5–6 mg/kg
Bupivacaine, ropivacaine, *l*-bupivacaine	2.5–3 mg/kg

[a]Large doses of local anesthetic are used infrequently during image-guided injections in pain medicine; however, doses nearing toxicity are used during certain blocks (e.g., celiac plexus block).

Table 4–4	
Approximate Equivalent Glucocorticoid Oral Dosages Established by Laboratory Assays	
Drug	**Equivalent Dose (mg)**
Cortisone	25
Hydrocortisone	20
Prednisolone	5
Prednisone	5
Methylprednisolone	4
Triamcinolone	4
Dexamethasone	0.75
Betamethasone	0.6

From ASHP Staff. *AHFS Drug Information Handbook 2004.* Bethesda, MD: American Society of Health-System Pharmacists; 2004:2,897, with permission.

cous and can be difficult to inject through small-bore needles. Care should be taken to use interlocking extension tubing and syringes to avoid sudden disconnections and splattering of personnel with the neurolytic solution.

Phenol has local anesthetic properties at lower concentrations and is neurolytic at higher concentrations. Concentrations below 5% cause protein denaturation, whereas higher concentrations produce protein coagulation and segmental demyelination. Poorly myelinated and unmyelinated nociceptive fibers are destroyed at concentrations of 5% to 6%, whereas higher concentrations cause axonal damage, spinal cord infarction, arachnoiditis, and meningitis. In contrast to alcohol, there is little or no pain on injection of phenol. The degree of neural blockade following injection of phenol is maximal in the first hours after injection and tends to subside somewhat thereafter. Large systemic doses of phenol (>8.5 g) cause effects similar to those seen with local anesthetic overdose: generalized seizures and cardiovascular collapse. Clinical doses up to 1,000 mg are unlikely to cause serious toxicity.

Ethyl Alcohol

Absolute (>98% concentration) ethyl alcohol is available commercially in 1- or 5-mL vials specifically for therapeutic neurolysis. Unlike phenol, alcohol injects readily through small-bore needles. Phenol causes intense pain when injected perineurally and must be preceded with local anesthetic or mixed directly with local anesthetic for injection to be tolerable to the patient.

Alcohol in concentrations above 33% results in extraction of cholesterol, phospholipids, and cerebrosides from neural tissue and precipitation of lipoproteins and mucoproteins. Alcohol produces nonselective destruction of neural tissue. The degree of neural blockade increases over the first several days following neurolysis with alcohol. Intravascular injection of 30 mL of 100% ethanol will result in a blood ethanol level well above the legal limit for intoxication but below

Table 4–5

Duration of Suppression of the Hypothalamic-Pituitary-Adrenal Axis Following Intramuscular Administration of Several Commercially Available Steroid Preparations

Drug	Brand Name (How Supplied)	IM Dose (mg)	Duration of HPA Axis Suppression
Triamcinolone acetonide	Kenalog (10 and 40 mg/mL)	40–80	2–4 wk
Triamcinolone diacetate	Aristocort Intralesional (25 mg/mL) Aristocort Forte (40 mg/mL)	50	1 wk
Betamethasone sodium phosphate/ betamethasone acetate suspension	Celestone Soluspan (betamethasone 6 mg/mL: betamethasone sodium phosphate 3 mg/mL and betamethasone acetate 3 mg/mL)	9	1 wk
Methylprednisolone acetate	Depo-Medrol (20, 40, or 80 mg/mL)	40–80	4–8 d

Table 4–6

Adverse Reactions Associated with Parenteral Glucocorticoid Administration

Body System	Adverse Reaction
Cardiovascular	Thromboembolism Thrombophlebitis Aggravation of hypertension
Dermatologic	Hyperpigmentation or hypopigmentation Subcutaneous fat atrophy Petechiae and ecchymoses
Central nervous system	Steroid psychoses Headache
Endocrine	Amenorrhea/menstrual abnormalities Hyperglycemia Increased insulin requirements in diabetics
Electrolyte disturbance	Sodium and fluid retention Hypokalemia Exacerbation of chronic congestive heart failure Peripheral edema
Gastrointestinal	Peptic ulcer with perforation and hemorrhage
Musculoskeletal	Steroid myopathy Osteoporosis Aseptic necrosis of femoral and humeral heads Spontaneous fractures
Miscellaneous	Anaphylactoid/hypersensitivity reactions

Data from *Drug Facts and Comparisons*. St. Louis, MO: Wolters Kluwer Health; 2005.

danger of severe alcohol toxicity. Alcohol is intensely inflammatory and has been associated with persistent or worsened pain and neuritis, particularly following peripheral neurolysis. This is believed to be caused by partial nerve injury during neurolysis.

SUGGESTED READINGS

Adrenocortical steroids. In: *Drug Facts and Comparisons*. St. Louis, MO: Wolters Kluwer Health; February 2002:319–325.

ASHP Staff. *AHFS Drug Information 2004*. Bethesda, MD: American Society of Health-System Pharmacists; 2004:2,892–2,919.

Brown DL. *Atlas of Regional Anesthesia*. 2nd ed. Philadelphia: WB Saunders; 1999:1–7.

Patt RB, Cousins MJ. Techniques for neurolytic neural blockade. In: Cousins MJ, Bridenbough PO, eds. *Neural Blockade in Clinical Anesthesia and Management of Pain*. 3rd ed. Philadelphia: JB Lippincott; 1998:1,007–1,062.

Viscomi CM. Pharmacology of local anesthetics. In: Rathmell JP, Neal JM, Viscomi CV, eds. *Requisites in Anesthesiology: Regional Anesthesia*. Philadelphia: Elsevier Health Sciences; 2004:13–24.

SPINAL INJECTION TECHNIQUES

Interlaminar Epidural Injection

Overview

Epidural injection has long been used to produce surgical anesthesia for operative procedures on the trunk, abdomen, and lower extremities. In recent years, epidural catheters have been left in place more frequently after major surgery to provide postoperative analgesia for several days. The more common use of epidural injection in the pain clinic is to place steroids into the epidural space, where they spread to bathe the exiting nerve roots to either side of midline. The rationale for injecting steroids is that they suppress inflammation in the nerve and adjacent soft tissues, which is believed to be the basis for radicular pain. The epidural space is entered from the posterior aspect near the midline, where a needle is advanced into the epidural space between adjacent vertebral laminae. This most common approach to the epidural space has been termed the "interlaminar approach." Identification of the epidural space requires familiarity with the loss-of-resistance (LOR) technique, which is described in detail later in this section. Using this technique, the epidural space is identified by the sudden LOR to injection as a needle passes from the interspinous ligament between adjacent spinous processes through the ligamentum flavum and into the low-resistance epidural space. Although anesthesiologists have used epidural anesthesia and analgesia for many years, more recently, pain practitioners have been moving toward use of the transforaminal route for placing steroids near an inflamed nerve root. The rationale for using a transforaminal route of injection, rather than an interlaminar route, is that the injectate is delivered directly to the target nerve. This ensures that the medication reaches the target area in maximum concentration at the site of the suspected pathology.

Anatomy

Bony Anatomy of the Vertebrae and Spinal Column

The structure of the vertebrae is distinct in the cervical, thoracic, and lumbar regions (Fig. 5-1). A typical vertebra consists of a spinous process that melds into bilateral laminae. The epidural space lies anterior to the laminae, and is bordered laterally by the pedicles and anteriorly by the vertebral body. Access to the epidural space is through the space between adjacent laminae (the "interlaminar" space). The superior and inferior articular processes of the facet joints lie posterolaterally over the junction between the laminae and the pedicles, and provide the lateral articulating surfaces between adjacent vertebrae. The sacral hiatus is the area where the fifth sacral vertebra (S5) lacks a spinous process and laminae posteriorly (Fig. 5-2). The two sacral cornua lie on either side of the sacral hiatus and cephalad to the coccyx.

Individual vertebral components can affect epidural block technique. The spinous processes vary in their degree of angulation at the various vertebral levels (Fig. 5-3). In the cervical and lumbar regions, the spinous process attaches to the lamina nearly horizontally, thus facilitating a midline perpendicular approach to the neuraxis. Conversely, the midthoracic (T5 to T9) spinous processes are acutely angulated to such an extent that paramedian approaches are much easier than those performed in the midline. High (T1 to T4) and low (T10 to T12) thoracic spinous processes are intermediate in their orientation, and are thus amenable to either an acutely angulated midline or a paramedian approach. The laminae become more vertically oriented as one progresses caudally; therefore, "walking off" the lamina is associated with progressively deeper needle placement from superior to inferior in the thoracic region. This also accounts for the more shallow depth on entering the lumbar region.

Surface landmarks can assist in identifying the approximate vertebral interspace (Table 5-1). In most humans, the C7 spinous process (the vertebrae prominens) is the most noticeable midline structure at the posterior neck base. A line drawn between the inferior angles of the scapulae identifies the T7 spinous process, whereas a line drawn between the iliac crests crosses the tip of the L4 spinous

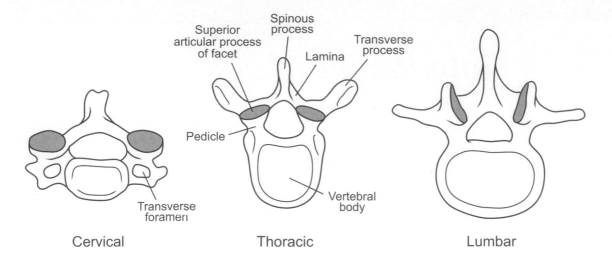

Figure 5-1.
Anatomy of the cervical, thoracic, and lumbar vertebrae.

process or the L4/L5 interspace. The spinal cord generally terminates at the L2 level, and the dural sac ends at S2 (the level of the posterior-superior iliac spines). The tip of an equilateral triangle drawn between the posterior-superior iliac spines and directed caudally overlies the sacral cornua and sacral hiatus.

Anatomy of the Epidural Space

Just as the bony structure of the vertebrae varies from the cervical to the sacral levels, so does the anatomy of the epidural space. The epidural space extends from the foramen magnum to the sacrococcygeal ligament. It is filled with epidural fat, a robust venous plexus, and loose areolar tissue. These contents are not as prominent in the thoracic and cervical space as in the lumbar region, where epidural veins are at their largest diameter. The ligamentum flavum is a structure of variable thickness and completeness that defines the posterolateral soft-tissue boundaries of the epidural space. Because the leatherlike consistency of the ligamentum flavum resists active expulsion of fluid from a syringe, loss of this resistance is valuable in signaling entry into the epidural space. The ligament's structure is steeply arched and tentlike, so much so that the lateral reflection may be up to 1 cm deeper than at the midline.

In the cervical and thoracic epidural spaces, the ligamentum flavum often does not fuse in the midline, which can become problematic during LOR techniques. When the dense ligamentum flavum is absent in the midline, it is possible to enter the epidural space without ever sensing significant resistance to injection. The ligamentum flavum is thickest at the lumbar and thoracic levels and thinnest at the cervical level. Its thickness also diminishes at the cephalad aspect of each interlaminar space and as the ligamentum flavum tapers off laterally. The epidural space itself progressively narrows in anterior-posterior (AP) dimension from the lumbar level (5 to 6 mm) to the thoracic level (3 to 5 mm), and is narrowest at the C3-to-C6 levels (2 mm). Because the spinal cord typically terminates at the L2 level, unintentional needle puncture of the dura below this level encounters free-floating filum terminale, rather than a fixed spinal cord. The posterior epidural space is narrow at cervical and thoracic levels, thus when the epidural space is entered, the needle tip lies in close proximity to the spinal cord.

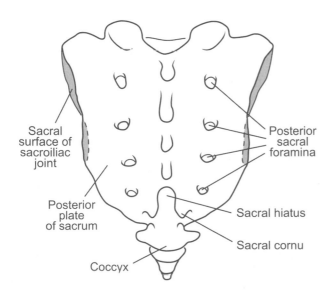

Figure 5-2.
Anatomy of the posterior sacrum and coccyx.

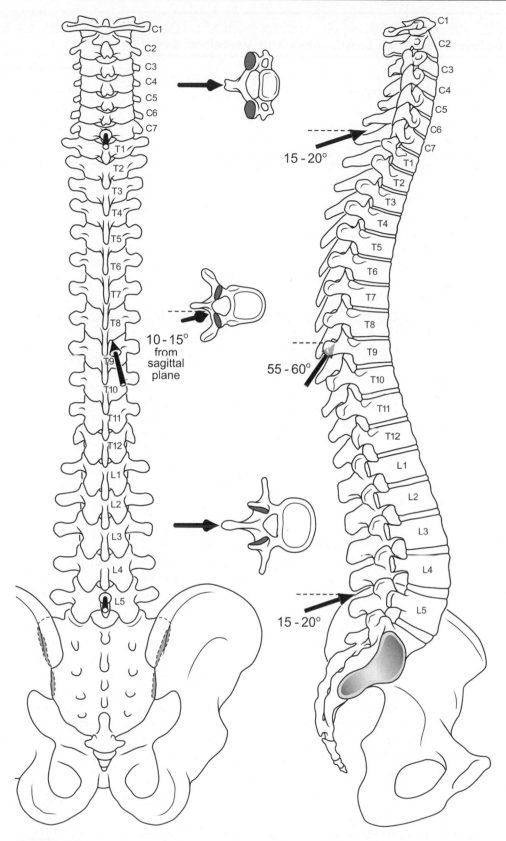

Figure 5-3.
Anatomy of the vertebral column. The most prominent spinous process at the base of the neck is C7 in most humans (the vertebrae prominens). Note that the angle of the spinous processes changes dramatically from cervical to lumbar levels, with the steepest angle in the midthoracic region. The approximate plane of needle entry for interlaminar epidural injection is shown for cervical, thoracic, and lumbar levels.

Table 5–1
Correlation Between Surface Landmarks and Vertebral Levels

Surface Landmark	Approximate Vertebral Level
Most prominent spinous process at base of neck (vertebra prominens)	C7 spinous process
Inferior angle of scapula	T7 spinous process
Superior margin of iliac crest	L4 spinous process or L4/L5 interspace
Posterior-Superior iliac spine	S2, termination of the dural sac
Inferior tip of equilateral triangle between posterior-superior iliac spines	Sacral hiatus

Above C7 to T1 and at intermittent areas along the posterior spinal canal, the epidural space is best described as a potential space that is easily dilated by injection of anesthetic solutions. Distribution of solutions within the epidural space is not uniform, especially as distance from the injection site increases. Rather, solutions spread along various routes as determined by small, low-resistance channels that exist between the epidural fat and veins. Nevertheless, solutions flow preferentially along the spinal nerve root sheaths because the only significant barrier to epidural flow appears to be the posterior longitudinal ligament, which serves to further direct anesthetic solutions toward the nerve roots. In patients who have undergone previous spinal surgery, scarring of the posterior epidural space is common, and the flow of injected solutions is less predictable.

Loss-of-Resistance Technique

Anesthesiologists learn to identify the epidural space "blindly" without the help of fluoroscopic guidance. This is accomplished using the LOR technique. Even when radiographic guidance is available, the LOR technique is still needed to identify the epidural space. Image guidance can help direct the needle toward the midline, between laminae, but neither AP nor lateral images can identify the precise location of the epidural space. The LOR technique is identical in the cervical, thoracic, and lumbar regions. After the skin and subcutaneous tissue have been anesthetized with a small volume of local anesthetic, an epidural needle is seated in the interspinous ligament, advancing 2 to 3 cm from the skin's surface (the most common type remains the 18- or 20-gauge Touhy needle; see Fig. 1-4). A syringe containing air or saline is then attached to the needle. Many practitioners prefer a 10-mL syringe containing 1 to 3 mL of isotonic saline and a small (~0.5 mL) bubble of air (Fig. 5-4A). The needle shaft is then grasped by the thumb and index finger of the non-dominant hand and advanced 1 to 2 mm at a time, while the first three fingers of the dominant hand are used to place gentle steady or intermittent pressure on the plunger of the syringe to test for resistance to injection as the needle is advanced toward the epidural space. The small bubble in the syringe is more compressible than the saline and

serves to visually reinforce the degree of resistance felt with each push on the syringe's plunger. As the needle tip traverses the ligamentum flavum and enters the dorsal epidural space, there is a discreet LOR to injection, and the saline exits the syringe to the epidural space. Also, because there is very low resistance to injection, the air bubble is no longer compressed (Fig. 5-4B).

Patient Selection

The most common indication for epidural injection in the pain clinic is to place corticosteroid adjacent to an inflamed nerve root that is causing radicular symptoms. Nerve root inflammation may stem from an acutely herniated intervertebral disc causing nerve root irritation or other causes of nerve root impingement such as isolated foraminal stenosis due to spondylitic spurring of the bony margins of the foramen. Epidural steroid injection is also used to treat symptoms of neurogenic claudication associated with spinal stenosis (stenosis of the central spinal canal). There are no scientific guidelines or any body of scientific literature to help choose between the interlaminar route and the transforaminal route for epidural injection of steroids, and each has unique complications. The spread of injectate during interlaminar injection, particularly when volumes of 5 mL or more are used, will often extend to both sides of midline and bathe the exiting nerve roots at the interspace of injection and at several adjacent interspaces. Thus, in those patients who present with bilateral radicular symptoms due to a midline disc herniation or neurogenic claudication in both legs due to central canal stensosis, it seems logical (if yet unproven) that interlaminar injection would be more likely to get the steroid solution to the target sites of nerve root irritation.

Cervical Epidural Injection

Positioning

The patient lies prone, facing the table, with a small headrest under the forehead to allow for air flow between the table and the patient's nose and mouth (Fig. 5-5). The c-arm is rotated 15 to 20 degrees caudally from the axial plane without any oblique angulation. This allows for good visualization

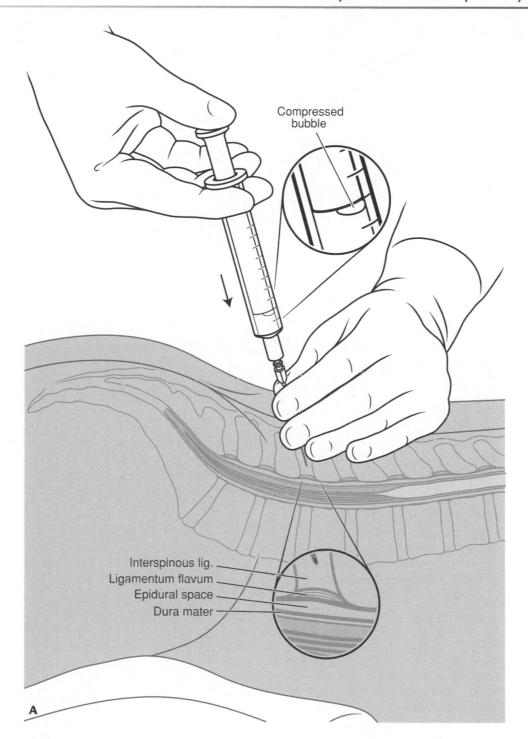

Compressed
bubble

Interspinous lig.
Ligamentum flavum
Epidural space
Dura mater

A

Figure 5-4.
The loss-of-resistance technique for identification of the epidural space using an interlaminar approach. **A:** The needle is seated in the interspinous ligament, and a syringe containing 1 to 3 mL of preservative-free saline and a small (~0.5 mL) air bubble is attached to the needle. The shaft of the needle is grasped firmly with the nondominant hand and intermittent or continuous light pressure is applied to the syringe plunger with the dominant hand. **B:** As the needle passes through the ligamentum flavum and into the epidural space, there is a sudden decrease or "loss" of resistance to injection. The air bubble in the syringe expands, and the saline in the syringe flows into the epidural space. Note the close proximity of the posterior surface of the dural sac; advancing the needle just a few additional millimeters will result in dural puncture and intrathecal location of the needle tip.

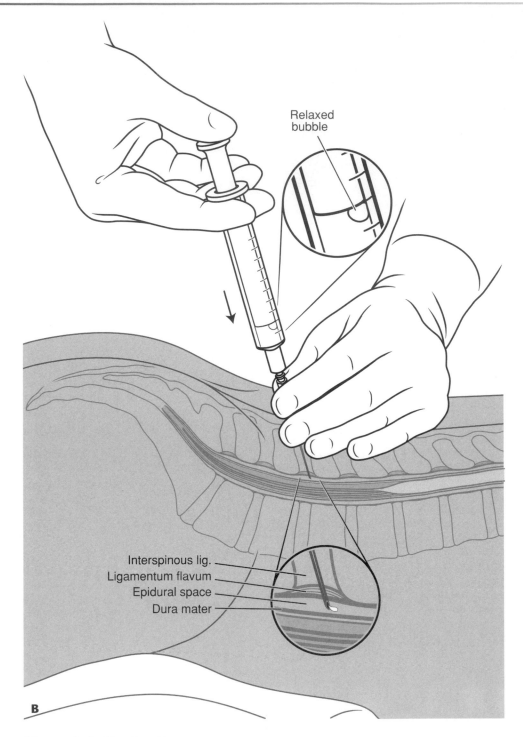

Relaxed
bubble

Interspinous lig.
Ligamentum flavum
Epidural space
Dura mater

B

Figure 5-4. *(Continued)*

of the interlaminar space and needle advancement between adjacent spinous processes (Figs. 5-6 and 5-7)

Block Technique

The skin and subcutaneous tissues overlying the interspace where the block is to be carried out are anesthetized with 1 to 2 mL of 1% lidocaine. The cervical interspaces with the largest interlaminar distance are typically found at C6/C7 and C7/T1. Because of the ease of entry, many practitioners will place the needle via one of these larger interspaces, regardless of the level of pathology, and rely on the flow of steroid in the epidural space to reach the level of pathology. The same technique can be carried out at all cervical interspaces at C3/C4 and below; interlaminar injection at the C2/C3 level and higher has not been described. An 18- or

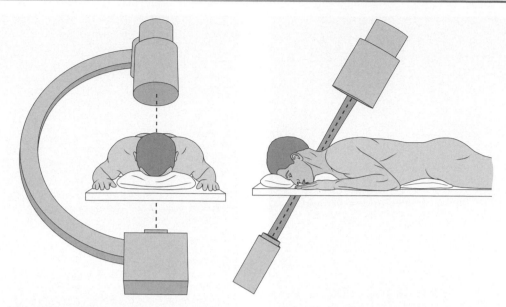

Figure 5-5.
Position for interlaminar cervical epidural injection. The patient is placed prone with a small headrest under the forehead to allow for air flow between the table and the patient's nose and mouth. The c-arm is angled 15 to 20 degrees caudally from the axial plane.

20-gauge Touhy needle is placed through the skin and advanced several centimeters until it is firmly seated in the interspinous ligament. An AP image is then taken, and the needle is redirected toward midline (see Fig. 5-7). A syringe containing 1 to 3 mL of preservative-free saline is attached to the needle, and the needle is slowly advanced in 1- to 2-mm increments until LOR occurs. Repeat images taken after every 0.5 to 1 cm of needle advancement will ensure the needle direction does not stray from midline. A firm grasp of the anatomy of adjacent structures and the proximity of the spinal cord are essential during cervical interlaminar epidural injection (Fig. 5-8). After the needle tip enters the epidural space, the position is confirmed by injecting 1 to 1.5 mL of nonionic radiographic contrast (iohexol 180 mg per mL), and contrast spread is verified in the AP and lateral planes. Lateral imaging of the cervicothoracic junction and

low cervical spine is hindered by the adjacent structures of the torso and arms (Fig. 5-9). A second lateral image taken just above the shoulders is often much simpler to interpret when trying to confirm epidural contrast flow (Fig. 5-10). Digital subtraction technology can also be extremely useful in ensuring injectate has spread to the level of pathology (Fig. 5-11). Once epidural needle position has been confirmed, a solution containing steroid diluted in preservative-free saline (80 mg of methyl prednisolone acetate or the equivalent diluted in 5 mL total volume) is injected, and the needle is removed.

Complications

Dural puncture with subsequent postdural puncture headache can occur during cervical interlaminar epidural

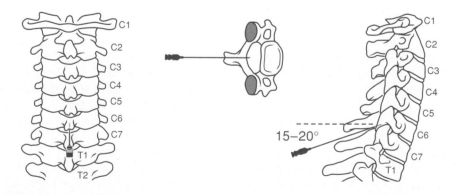

Figure 5-6.
Position and angle of needle entry for cervical interlaminar epidural injection. An 18- or 20-gauge Touhy needle is advanced in the midline with 15 to 20 degrees of caudad angulation from the axial plane parallel to the spinous processes.

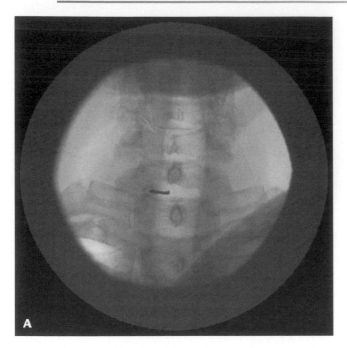
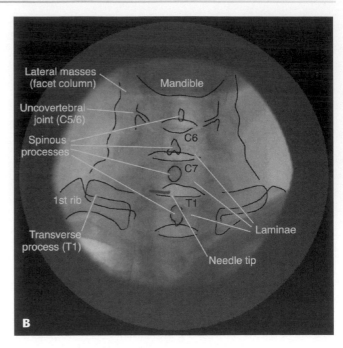

Figure 5-7.
Anterior-Posterior radiographs of the cervical spine during cervical interlaminar injection.
A: An 18-gauge Touhy needle is in position between the C7 and T1 laminae and spinous
processes. The needle tip is directly between spinous processes, whereas the hub is to the
left of the image. **B:** Labeled image.

injection. Although cervical epidural blood patch using a
small volume of autologous blood has been described,
most practitioners will manage postdural puncture
headache following cervical epidural injection conservatively with fluids and oral analgesics. The incidence of
headache following cervical dural puncture is lower than
that following lumbar puncture, likely due to the dimin-
ished column of cerebrospinal fluid (CSF) cephalad to the
point of dural puncture. Direct trauma to the spinal cord
with catastrophic consequences (quadriplegia) has also
been described, particularly in heavily sedated patients.
The level of sedation during this procedure should allow
for direct conversation between the practitioner and the
patient to ensure that the patient can report contact with
neural elements before significant traumatic injury
occurs. Caution should also be taken to avoid interlaminar epidural injection at any level where there is effacement of the epidural space (e.g., complete effacement of
the epidural space and the CSF column surrounding the
spinal cord within the thecal sac occurs in high-grade
spinal stenosis, particularly that due to a large central or
paramedian disc herniation). As with interlaminar
epidural injection at all vertebral levels, epidural bleeding
or infection can occur. Epidural hematoma or abscess can
lead to significant spinal cord compression. Interlaminar
injection should be avoided or postponed in those receiving anticoagulants.

Thoracic Epidural Injection

Positioning.

The patient lies prone, with the head turned to one side
(Fig. 5-12). The c-arm is rotated 40 to 50 degrees caudally
from the axial plane without any oblique angulation. This
allows for good visualization of the interlaminar space and
needle advancement between adjacent spinous processes
(Figs. 5-13 and 5-14).

Block Technique

The skin and subcutaneous tissues approximately 1 cm lateral and 1 cm caudal to the interspace where the block is to
be carried out are anesthetized with 1 to 2 mL of 1% lidocaine. An 18- or 20-gauge Touhy needle is placed through
the skin and advanced several centimeters until it is firmly
seated in tissue. An AP image is then taken and the needle
is redirected toward the inferior margin of the lamina that
bounds the inferior aspect of the interspace that is to be
entered near the junction of the spinous process and the
lamina (see Fig. 5-14). Although a midline approach can be
used at low thoracic levels, the spinous processes are angled
too steeply to allow for true coaxial needle placement at the
midthoracic levels. Thus, the needle is directed toward the
margin of the lamina. The needle is advanced in 3- to 4-mm
increments and repeat images are taken. Care must be taken

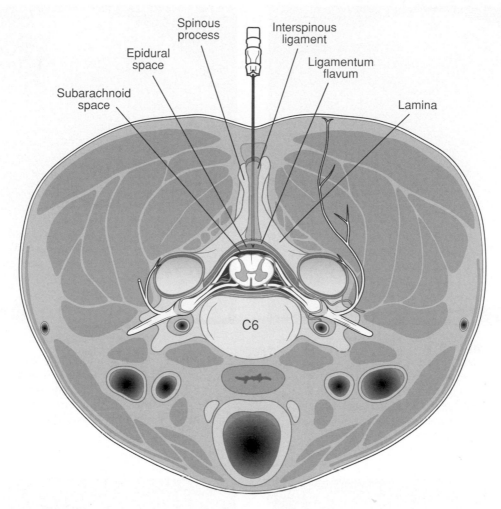

Figure 5-8.
Axial diagram of interlaminar cervical epidural injection. The epidural needle is advanced in the midline between spinous processes and traverses the ligamentum flavum to enter the dorsal epidural space in the midline. The normal epidural space is approximately 2 mm wide (from the ligamentum flavum to the dura mater in the axial plane). Note the proximity of the underlying spinal cord during cervical epidural injection.

to keep the needle tip over the margin of the lamina until bone is gently contacted. The periosteum should then be anesthetized with an additional 1 mL of 1% lidocaine and a syringe containing 1 to 3 mL of preservative-free saline attached to the needle. The needle is slowly advanced over the superior margin of the lamina and into the interlaminar space in 1- to 2-mm increments until LOR occurs. Because the needle is unlikely to lie within the interspinous ligament when using a paramedian approach, there will be little resistance to injection until the needle enters the interlaminar space and traverses the ligamentum flavum. A firm grasp of the anatomy of adjacent structures and the proximity of the spinal cord are essential during thoracic interlaminar epidural injection (Fig. 5-15). After the needle tip enters the epidural space, the position is confirmed by injecting 1 to 1.5 mL of nonionic radiographic contrast (iohexol 180 mg per mL), and contrast spread is verified in

the AP and lateral planes. Lateral imaging of the thoracic spine is hindered by the overlying structures of the thorax (Fig. 5-16). Once epidural needle position has been confirmed, a solution containing steroid diluted in preservative-free saline (80 mg of methyl prednisolone acetate or the equivalent diluted in 5 mL total volume) is injected, and the needle is removed.

Complications

Dural puncture with subsequent postdural puncture headache can occur during thoracic interlaminar epidural injection. Although thoracic epidural blood patch using a small volume of autologous blood has been described, most practitioners will manage postdural puncture headache following thoracic epidural injection conservatively with fluids and oral analgesics. The incidence of

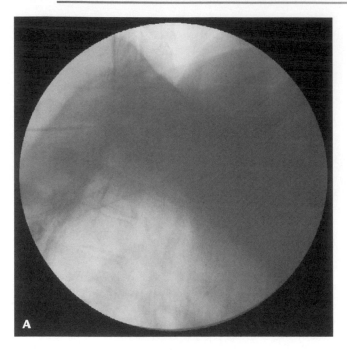
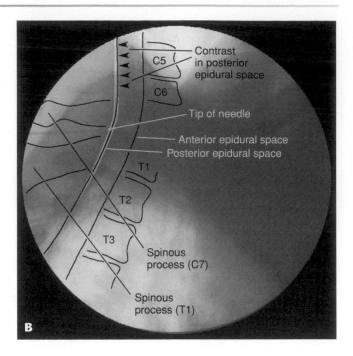

Figure 5-9.

Lateral radiograph of the cervical spine near the cervicothoracic junction during interlaminar cervical epidural injection. **A:** A Touhy needle is in place in the C7/T1 interspace extending to the dorsal epidural space. One and one-half milliliters of radiographic contrast has been injected and can be seen as a thin stripe toward the upper aspect of the image. Lateral radiographs near the cervicothoracic junction are difficult to interpret because of the overlying structures of the thorax and upper extremities. **B:** Labeled image.

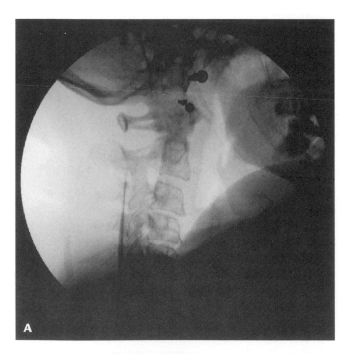
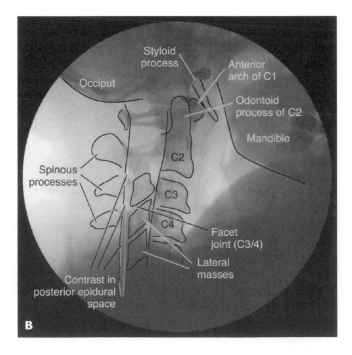

Figure 5-10.

Lateral radiograph of the upper cervical spine during interlaminar cervical epidural injection. **A:** Lateral radiograph of the superior cervical spine after injection of 1.5 mL of radiographic contrast at the C6/C7 level (see Fig. 5-9). The contrast can be seen as a thin stripe toward the posterior aspect of the spinal canal, adjacent to the anterior-most aspect of each spinous process. Although lateral radiographs near the cervicothoracic junction are difficult to interpret because of the overlying structures of the thorax and upper extremities, lateral radiographs of the superior cervical spine can be used to verify epidural placement. **B:** Labeled image.

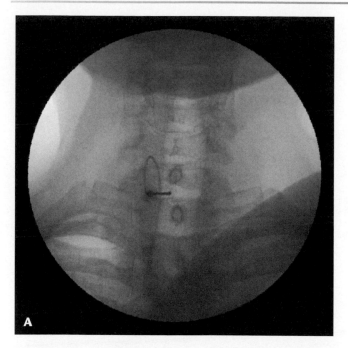
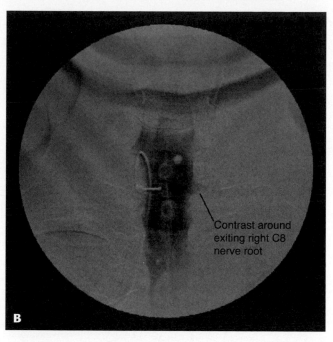

Contrast around
exiting right C8
nerve root

Figure 5-11.
Digital subtraction epidurogram following interlaminar cervical epidural steroid injection.
A: Anterior-Posterior radiograph showing the epidural needle in final position for contrast injection via flexible extension tubing. **B:** Final digital subtraction image following injection of 1.5 mL of radiographic contrast. Note the contrast spread nearly two vertebral levels above and below the level of injection and outlining the exiting nerve roots on both sides.

headache following thoracic dural puncture is high (50% or more of patients), approaching that following lumbar puncture. Direct trauma to the spinal cord with catastrophic consequences (quadriplegia) has also been described, particularly in heavily sedated patients. The level of sedation during this procedure should allow for direct con-versation between the practitioner and the patient to ensure the patient can report contact with neural elements before significant traumatic injury occurs. Caution should also be taken to avoid interlaminar epidural injection at any level where there is effacement of the epidural space (e.g., complete effacement of the epidural space and the

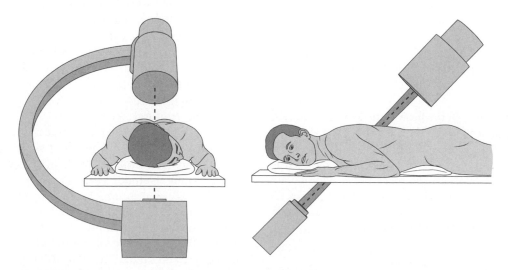

Figure 5-12.
Position for interlaminar thoracic epidural injection. The patient is placed prone with the head turned to one side. The c-arm is angled 40 to 50 degrees caudally from the axial plane.

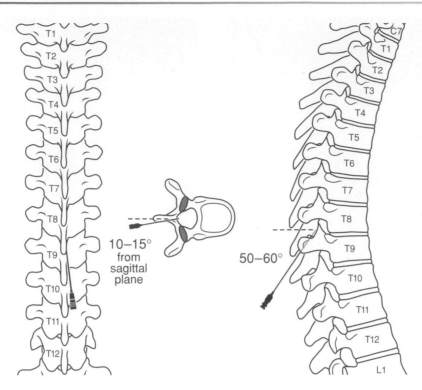

Figure 5-13.
Position and angle of needle entry for thoracic interlaminar epidural injection (paramedian approach). Starting approximately 1 cm below the interspace and 1 cm lateral to the spinous processes, an 18- or 20-gauge Touhy needle is advanced 10 to 15 degrees toward midline with 50 to 60 degrees of caudad angulation from the axial plane.

CSF column surrounding the spinal cord within the thecal sac occurs in high-grade spinal stenosis, particularly that due to a large central or paramedian disc herniation). As with interlaminar epidural injection at all vertebral levels, epidural bleeding or infection can occur. Epidural hematoma or abscess can lead to significant spinal cord compression. Interlaminar injection should be avoided or postponed in those receiving anticoagulants.

Lumbar Epidural Injection

Positioning

The patient lies prone with the head turned to one side (Fig. 5-17). A pillow is placed under the mid- and lower abdomen to reduce the lumbar lordosis and increase the separation between adjacent spinous processes. The c-arm is rotated 15 to 20 degrees caudally from the axial plane without any oblique angulation. This allows for good visualization of the interlaminar space and needle advancement between adjacent spinous processes (Figs. 5-18 and 5-19).

Block Technique

The skin and subcutaneous tissues overlying the interspace where the block is to be carried out are anesthetized with 1 to 2 mL of 1% lidocaine. An 18- or 20-gauge Touhy needle is placed through the skin and advanced 1 to 2 cm until it is firmly seated in the interspinous ligament. An AP image is then taken, and the needle is directed toward midline (see Fig. 5-19). A syringe containing 1 to 3 mL of preservative-free saline is attached to the needle, and the needle is slowly advanced in 1- to 2-mm increments until LOR occurs. Repeat images taken after every 0.5 to 1 cm of needle advancement will ensure the needle direction does not stray from midline. A firm knowledge of the anatomy of adjacent structures, as well as the proximity of the thecal sac and cauda equina, are essential during lumbar interlaminar epidural injection (Fig. 5-20). After the needle tip enters the epidural space, the position is confirmed by injecting 1 to 1.5 mL of nonionic radiographic contrast (iohexol 180 mg per mL), and contrast spread is verified in the AP and lateral planes. Lateral imaging of the lower lumbar spine is hindered by the overlying iliac crests (Fig. 5-21); visualization can also be quite difficult in the obese patient. Once epidural needle position has been confirmed, a solution containing steroid diluted in preservative-free saline (80 mg of methylprednisolone acetate or the equivalent diluted in 5 to 10 mL total volume) is injected, and the needle is removed. When larger injectate volumes are used, the solution spreads extensively in both the anterior and posterior aspects of the epidural space

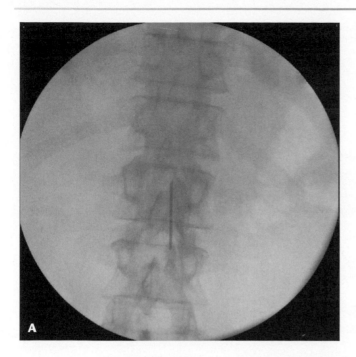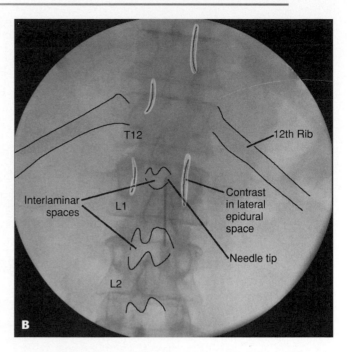

Figure 5-14.

Posterior-Anterior radiograph of the thoracic spine during thoracic interlaminar injection (paramedian approach). **A:** An 18-gauge Touhy needle is in position between the T12 and L1 laminae just to the right of midline. The needle should first be advanced, keeping the needle tip over the superior margin of the lamina bounding the inferior aspect of the interspace to be entered (in this example, the superior margin of the lamina of L1 to the right of midline). The needle is advanced until it gently touches the lamina where it joins with the spinous process. Using the paramedian approach, contacting the margin of lamina allows determination of depth before entering the interspace and starting loss-of-resistance (LOR) to identify the epidural space. This paramedian approach is often necessary at thoracic levels because of the steep angulation of the spinous processes. With the paramedian approach, the LOR technique is unreliable until the needle is seated within the ligamentum flavum; at more superficial levels, there is little resistance to injection. **B:** Labeled image.

(Figs. 5-22 and 5-23). In patients with significant lumbar pathology (e.g., a herniated intervertebral disc), the injectate will tend to follow the path of least resistance, often flowing toward the side opposite the pathology.

Complications

Dural puncture with subsequent postdural puncture headache can occur during lumbar interlaminar epidural injection. The incidence of unintentional dural puncture may be higher in those with previous lumbar surgery, due to scarring within the epidural space and adhesion of the dura to the posterior elements. Epidural blood patch using autologous blood is a safe and effective treatment that relieves the headache symptoms promptly in the majority of those who fail to improve after 24 to 48 hours of conservative treatment with fluids and oral analgesics. Direct trauma to the cauda equina or exiting nerve roots is unlikely during lumbar epidural injection

when disciplined use of radiographic guidance is employed to ensure the needle tip does not stray from the midline. The level of sedation during this procedure should allow for direct conversation between the practitioner and the patient to ensure the patient can report contact with neural elements before significant traumatic injury occurs. As with interlaminar epidural injection at all vertebral levels, epidural bleeding or infection can occur. Epidural hematoma or abscess can lead to significant spinal cord compression. Interlaminar injection should be avoided or postponed in those receiving anticoagulants.

Caudal Epidural Injection

Positioning

The patient lies prone with the head turned to one side (Fig. 5-24). The c-arm is rotated 20 to 30 degrees caudally

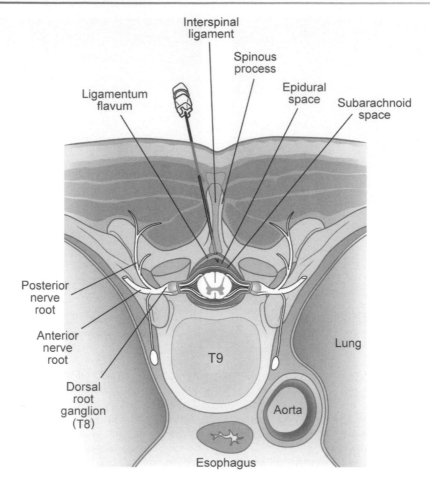

Figure 5-15.
Axial diagram of interlaminar thoracic epidural injection. The epidural needle is advanced toward the midline using a paramedian approach and traverses the ligamentum flavum to enter the dorsal epidural space in the midline. The normal epidural space is approximately 3 to 5 mm wide (from the ligamentum flavum to the dura mater in the axial plane). Note the proximity of the underlying spinal cord during thoracic epidural injection.

from the axial plane without any oblique angulation. This allows for good visualization of the sacrum, sacral hiatus, and coccyx (Figs. 5-25 and 5-26).

Block Technique

The sacral hiatus is identified radiographically (see Fig. 5-26) and the overlying skin and subcutaneous tissues are anesthetized with 1 to 2 mL of 1% lidocaine. The sacral hiatus can be quite difficult to visualize radiographically. The approximate location can be identified by palpating the paired sacral corneae in the midline, near the superior extent of the gluteal cleft. An 18- or 20-gauge Touhy needle can be used, but a smaller 22-gauge, 3.5-inch spinal needle is perfectly adequate. The needle is placed through the skin and advanced directly through the sacrococcygeal ligament. As the needle passes through the ligament, a distinct "pop" can be felt. Once the needle has passed through the sacrococcygeal ligament and

into the caudal spinal canal, the angle of the needle is decreased to lie closer to the plane of the sacrum, and the needle is advanced into the caudal canal an additional 1 to 2 cm. A firm grasp of the anatomy of the sacral hiatus and the caudal epidural space is essential during caudal epidural injection (Figs. 5-25 and 5-27). AP and lateral radiographs confirm the needle's position within the caudal epidural space (Figs. 5-26 and 5-28), the caudal epidural space is generously supplied with veins, and intravascular needle placement is confirmed by injecting 1 to 1.5 mL of nonionic radiographic contrast (iohexol 180 mg per mL) under live fluoroscopy. Once caudal epidural needle position has been confirmed, a solution containing steroid diluted in preservative-free saline (80 mg of methylprednisolone acetate or the equivalent diluted in at least 10 mL total volume) is injected, and the needle is removed. The caudal epidural space is distant from the usual sites of nerve root inflammation near the lumbosacral junction, thus a significant volume of injectate (at least 10 mL) is

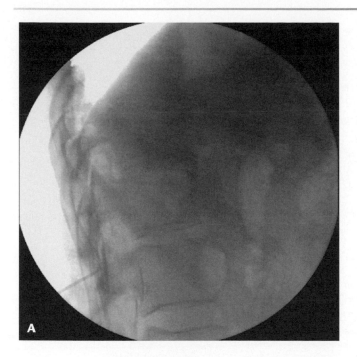
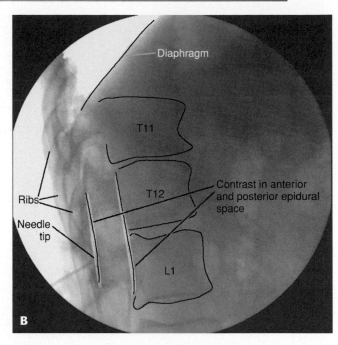

Figure 5-16.

Lateral radiograph of the thoracic spine during interlaminar thoracic epidural injection. **A:** A Touhy needle is in place in the T12/L1 interspace extending to the dorsal epidural space. One and one-half milliliters of radiographic contrast has been injected, and can be seen in the posterior epidural space near the tip of the needle and as a thin stripe along the anterior epidural space adjacent to the vertebral bodies. Lateral radiographs of the thoracic spine are difficult to interpret because of the overlying structures of the thorax and the air contrast of the overlying lung fields. **B:** Labeled image.

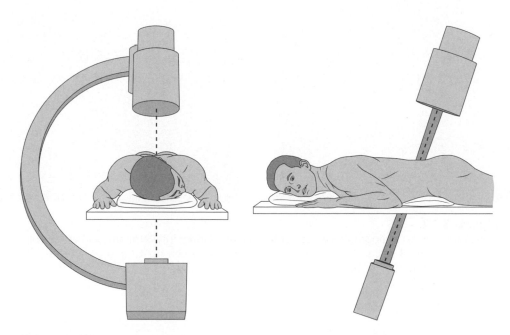

Figure 5-17.

Position for interlaminar lumbar epidural injection. The patient is placed prone with the head turned to one side. A pillow is placed under the mid- and lower abdomen to reduce the lumbar lordosis and increase the distance between adjacent spinous processes. The c-arm is angled 15 to 20 degrees caudally from the axial plane.

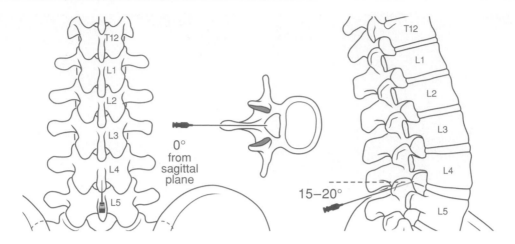

Figure 5-18.
Position and angle of needle entry for lumbar interlaminar epidural injection. An 18- or 20-gauge Touhy needle is advanced in the midline with 15 to 20 degrees of caudad angulation from the axial plane parallel to the spinous processes.

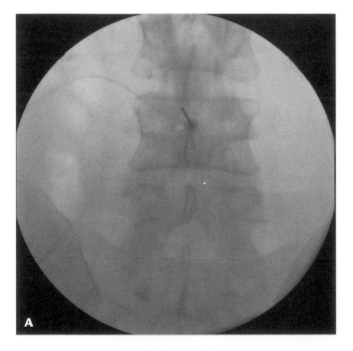
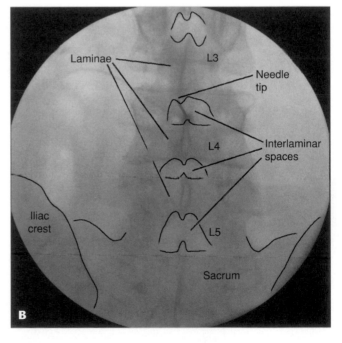

Figure 5-19.
Anterior-Posterior radiograph of the lumbar spine during interlaminar lumbar epidural injection. **A:** An 18-gauge Touhy needle is in position between the L3 and L4 laminae with the tip extending just to the left of midline. **B:** Labeled image.

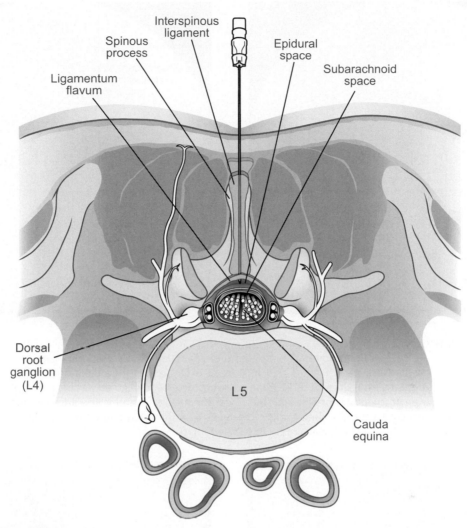

Figure 5-20.
Axial diagram of interlaminar lumbar epidural injection. The epidural needle is advanced in the midline between adjacent spinous processes to traverse the ligamentum flavum and enter the dorsal epidural space in the midline. The normal epidural space is approximately 4 to 6 mm wide (from the ligamentum flavum to the dura mater in the axial plane). Note the proximity of the underlying cauda equina during lumbar epidural injection.

usually required to affect spread to the level of the lumbosacral junction.

Complications

Dural puncture with subsequent postdural puncture headache can occur during caudal epidural injection, but it should occur only if the needle is advanced several centimeters or more cephalad within the caudal spinal canal. The thecal sac extends to the level of approximately S2, and the position can be approximated by palpating the adjacent posterior-superior iliac spines, which lie at approximately the same level. Direct trauma to the cauda equina or the exiting nerve roots is unlikely with the caudal approach. As with interlaminar epidural injection at all vertebral levels, epidural bleeding or infection can occur. Epidural hematoma or abscess can lead to significant compression of the cauda equina. Caudal epidural injection should be avoided or postponed in those receiving anticoagulants.

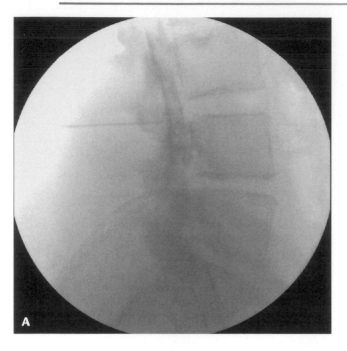
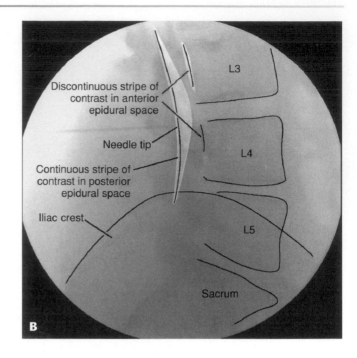

Figure 5-21.

Lateral radiograph of the lumbar spine during interlaminar lumbar epidural injection. **A:** A Touhy needle is in place in the L3/L4 interspace extending to the dorsal epidural space. One and one-half milliliters of radiographic contrast has been injected, and can be seen as a thin stripe in the posterior epidural space near the needle tip and in the anterior epidural space adjacent to the vertebral bodies. Lateral radiographs of the lumbar spine are often hindered by the overlying iliac crests. **B:** Labeled image.

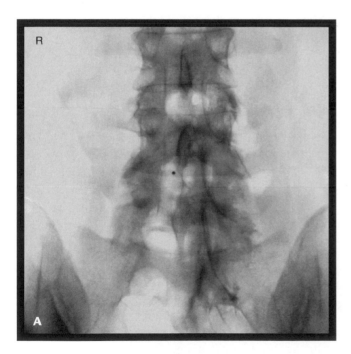
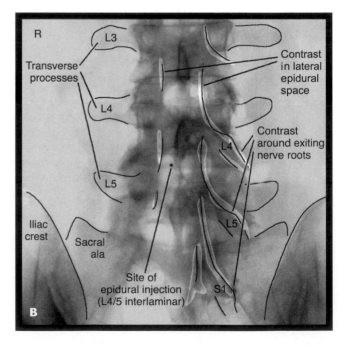

Figure 5-22.

Anterior-Posterior epidurogram of the lumbosacral spine. **A:** When larger volumes of injectate are used (in this image, 10 mL of contrast-containing solution), the injectate spreads extensively within the anterior and posterior epidural space and exits the intervertebral foramina, surrounding the exiting nerve roots. However, in the presence of significant obstruction to flow, as in this patient with a right L4/L5 disc herniation and compression of the exiting right L4 nerve root, the injectate often follows the path of least resistance, exiting the foramina on the side *opposite* from the disc herniation. **B:** Labeled image. (Adapted from Rathmell JP, Torian D, Song T. Lumbar epidurography. *Reg Anesth Pain Med*. 2000;25:542, with permission.)

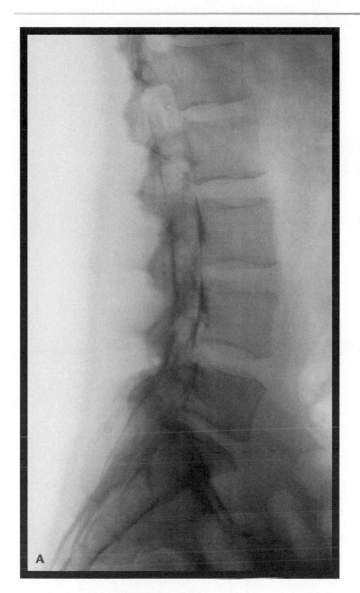

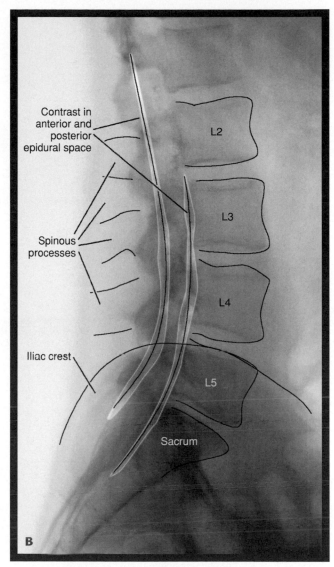

Figure 5-23.
A: Lateral epidurogram of the lumbosacral spine. When larger volumes of injectate are used (in this image, 10 mL of contrast-containing solution), the injectate spreads extensively within the anterior and posterior epidural space and has a characteristic "double line" or "railroad track" appearance. **B:** Labeled image. (Adapted from Rathmell JP, Torian D, Song T. Lumbar epidurography. *Reg Anesth Pain Med.* 2000;25:542, with permission.)

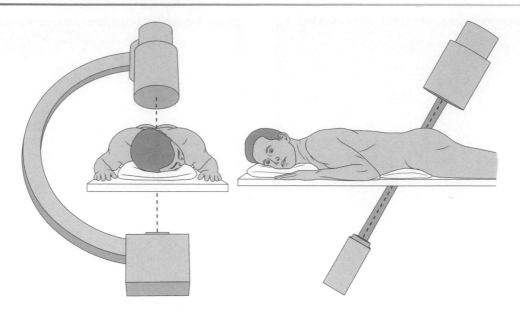

Figure 5-24.
Position for caudal epidural injection. The patient is placed prone with the head turned to one side. The c-arm is angled 20 to 30 degrees caudally from the axial plane.

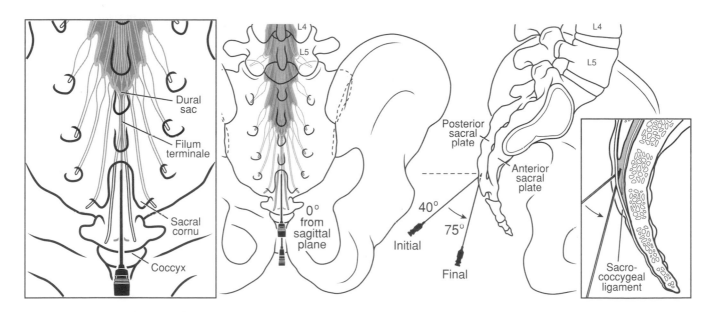

Figure 5-25.
Position and angle of needle entry for caudal epidural injection. A 22-gauge, 3.5-inch spinal needle (some practitioners prefer a 20-gauge Touhy needle) is advanced in the midline overlying the sacral hiatus. A distinct "pop" is felt as the needle tip passes through the sacrococcygeal ligament. The angle of the needle is then increased (to 75 degrees or more from the axial plane) to lie closer to the plane of the sacrum, and the needle tip is advanced an additional 1 to 2 cm into the sacral spinal canal. Note the inferior termination of the thecal sac at approximately S2.

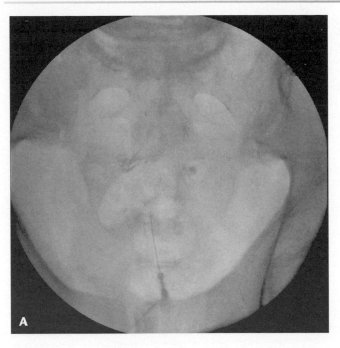
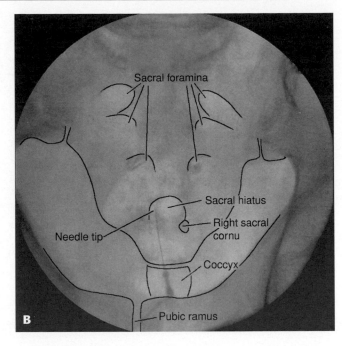

Figure 5-26.
Anterior-Posterior radiograph of the sacrum during caudal epidural injection. **A:** A 22-gauge spinal needle is in position through the sacral hiatus and directed toward the left of midline. **B:** Labeled image.

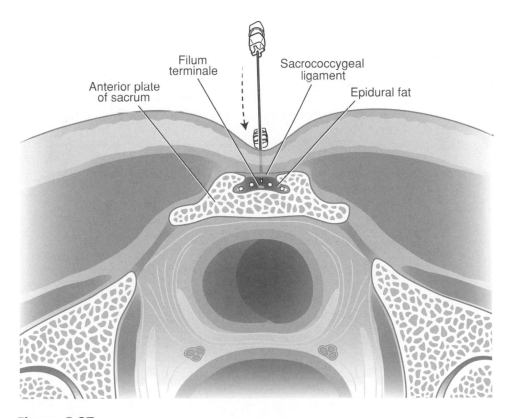

Figure 5-27.
Axial diagram of caudal epidural injection. The needle is advanced through the sacrococcygeal ligament. The angle is then increased to allow the needle to be advanced more cephalad within the epidural space.

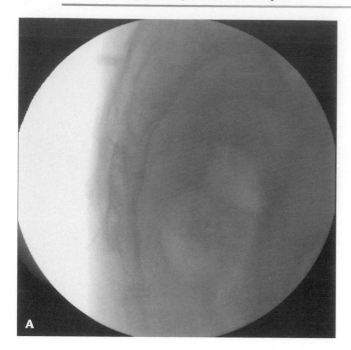
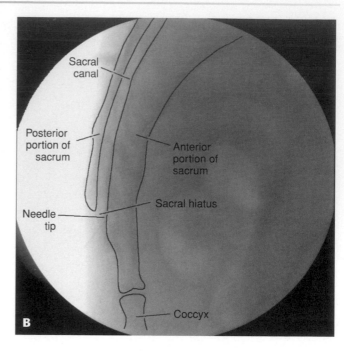

Figure 5-28.

Lateral radiograph of the sacrum during caudal epidural injection. **A:** A 22-gauge spinal needle is in place through the sacrococcygeal ligament. The tip of the needle is resting against the anterior plate of the sacrum. From this point, the needle angle should be brought into line with the axis of the caudal canal and advanced an additional 1 to 2 cm. **B:** Labeled image.

SUGGESTED READINGS

Abram SE. Treatment of lumbosacral radiculopathy with epidural steroids. *Anesthesiology.* 1999;91:1937–1941.

Abram SE, O'Connor TC. Complications associated with epidural steroid injections. *Reg Anesth.* 1996;21:149–162.

Brown DL. *Atlas of Regional Anesthesia.* 2nd ed. Philadelphia: WB Saunders; 1999:329–355.

Cousins MJ, Veering BT. Epidural neural blockade. In: Cousins MG, Bridenbaugh PO, eds. *Neural Blockade in Clinical Anesthesia and Management of Pain.* 3rd ed. Philadelphia: Lippincott-Raven; 1998:243–321.

Field J, Rathmell JP, Stephenson JH et al. Neuropathic pain following cervical epidural steroid injection. *Anesthesiology.* 2000;93:885–888.

Hogan QH. Epidural anatomy examined by cryomicrotome section. Influence of age, vertebral level, and disease. *Reg Anesth.* 1996;21:395–406.

Horlocker TT, Wedel DJ, Benzon H et al. Regional anesthesia in the anticoagulated patient: defining the risks. The second ASRA consensus conference on neuraxial anesthesia and anticoagulation. *Reg Anesth Pain Med.* 2003;28:172–197.

Mulligan KA, Rowlingson JC. Epidural steroids. *Curr Pain Headache Rep.* 2001;5:495–502.

Neal JM. Epidural anesthesia. In: Rathmell JP, Neal JM, Viscomi CV, eds. *Requisites in Anesthesiology: Regional Anesthesia.* Philadelphia: Elsevier Health Sciences, 2004:99–113.

Rathmell JP, Torian D, Song T. Lumbar epidurography. *Reg Anesth Pain Med.* 2000;25:540–545.

Weinstein SM, Herring SA: NASS. Lumbar epidural steroid injections. *Spine J.* 2003;3(3 Suppl):37S–44S.

CHAPTER 6

Transforaminal and Selective Nerve Root Injection

Overview

Selective nerve root injection and transforaminal epidural injection can be performed using similar techniques. Indeed, the distinction between the two techniques is questionable because the fascial sheath surrounding the exiting nerve roots is contiguous with the dura mater within the epidural space. A solution injected around an exiting nerve root may well enter the epidural space, regardless of whether the needle tip is advanced through the intervertebral foramen prior to injection. Nonetheless, many practitioners reserve the term "selective nerve root injection" for injections that are performed with the needle tip adjacent to the exiting nerve root, *outside* the intervertebral foramen, and the term "transforaminal injection" for injections that are performed with the needle tip *within* the intervertebral foramen. The rationale for injecting steroids is that they suppress inflammation of the nerve, which is believed to be the basis for radicular pain. The rationale for using a transforaminal route of injection rather than an interlaminar route is that the injectate is delivered directly onto the target nerve. This ensures the medication reaches the target area in maximum concentration at the site of the suspected pathology.

Cervical Transforaminal and Selective Nerve Root Injection

Anatomy

At typical cervical levels, the ventral and dorsal roots of the spinal nerves descend in the vertebral canal to form the spinal nerve in their intervertebral foramen. The foramen faces obliquely forward and lateral. Its roof and floor are formed by the pedicles of consecutive vertebrae. Its pos-terolateral wall is formed largely by the superior articular process of the lower vertebra, and in part by the inferior articular process of the upper vertebra and the capsule of the zygapophysial joint formed between the two articular processes. The anteromedial wall is formed by the lower end of the upper vertebral body, the uncinate process of the lower vertebra, and the posterolateral corner of the intervertebral disc. Immediately lateral to the external opening of the foramen, the vertebral artery rises closely in front of the articular pillars of the zygapophysial joint (Fig. 6-1). The spinal nerve, in its dural sleeve, lies in the lower half of the foramen. The upper half is occupied by epiradicular veins. The ventral ramus of the spinal nerve issues from the intervertebral foramen, passing forward and lateral onto the transverse process. In strict anatomic terms, what has been termed "selective nerve root injection" would be more precisely termed "selective spinal nerve injection," as the technique is carried out at the level of the spinal nerve, not the more proximal ventral and dorsal roots. However, the terms "selective nerve root injection" and "selective nerve root block" have permeated the published literature, and here we will use the widely accepted albeit innacurate terminology. Arterial branches arise from the vertebral arteries to supply the nerve roots (radicular arteries) or the spinal cord via the anterior and posterior spinal arteries (medullary arteries) (see Fig. 6-1). Medullary and radicular arterial branches may also arise from the deep or ascending cervical arteries and traverse through the entire length of the foramen adjacent to the spinal nerve (see Fig. 6-1), and it is these spinal segmental arteries that are at risk for penetration during cervical transforaminal injection.

Patient Selection

The most common indication for selective nerve root injection is to place corticosteroid adjacent to an inflamed nerve root that is causing radicular symptoms. Nerve root inflammation may stem from an acutely herniated intervertebral disc causing nerve root irritation or other causes of nerve root impingement, such as isolated foraminal stenosis due to spondylitic spurring of the bony margins of the foramen. Selective nerve root injection with local anesthetic has also been employed diagnostically to determine which nerve root is causing symptoms when pathology exists at multiple vertebral levels. This information can prove helpful in planning surgical intervention.

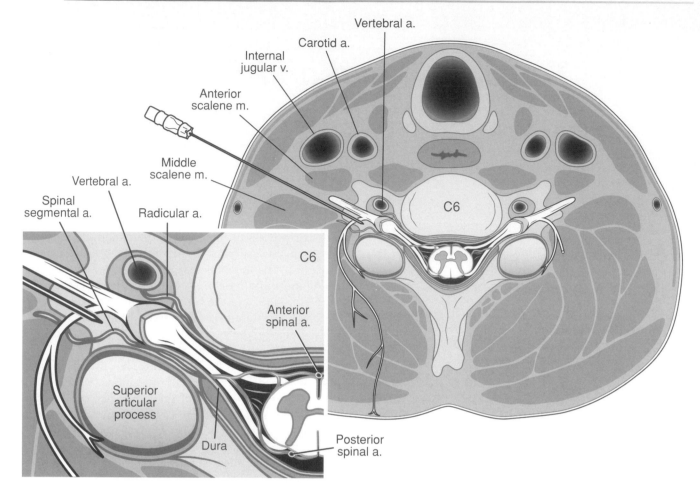

Figure 6-1.
Axial view of cervical transforaminal injection at the level of C6. The needle has been inserted along the axis of the foramen, and is illustrated in final position within the posterior aspect of the foramen. Insertion along this axis avoids the vertebral artery, which lies anterior to the foramen, and the exiting nerve root. Spinal segmental arteries arise from the deep or ascending cervical artery, enter the foramen at variable locations and often course through the foramen, penetrate the dura, and join the anterior or posterior spinal arteries that supply the spinal cord (*inset*). An arterial branch that joins the anterior spinal artery is termed a segmental "medullary" artery. Likewise, arterial branches arise variably from the vertebral artery to supply the nerve root itself (here a branch to the nerve root or "radicular" artery is illustrated); similar branches from the vertebral artery often penetrate the dura to join the anterior or posterior spinal artery. There is great anatomic variation in the vascular supply in this region. The anatomic variant illustrated is shown to demonstrate how a small artery that provides critical reinforcing blood supply to the spinal cord can be entered during cervical transforaminal injection. Injection of particulate steroid directly into one of these vessels can lead to catastrophic spinal cord injury. (Anatomic descriptions are based on cadaveric dissections carried out in our laboratory. Preliminary data appear in Hoeft MA, Rathmell JP, Monsey RD et al. *Anatomy of the Cervical Radicular Arteries: Implications for Cervical Transforaminal Injection*. Presented at the annual fall meeting of the American Society of Regional Anesthesia and Pain Medicine, Phoenix, AZ, November 11–14, 2004.)

Positioning

The patient lies supine, facing directly forward (Fig. 6-2). The c-arm is rotated 45 to 65 degrees lateral oblique until the neural foramina are clearly visualized (Fig. 6-3). The patient may also be asked to rotate the head away from the side of injection. Although this facilitates access to the side of the neck, the neural foramina and bony elements of the cervical spine will no longer be aligned. This may prove confusing to the inexperienced practitioner.

Block Technique

A 25-gauge, 2-inch blunt-tipped needle is sufficient in length for all but the most obese patients. To avoid the vertebral artery and the exiting nerve root, the needle is

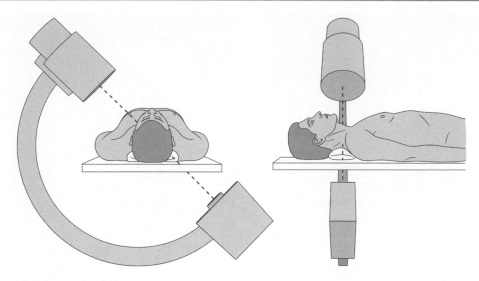

Figure 6-2.

Patient position for cervical transforaminal injection. The patient is positioned supine with c-arm axis rotated obliquely 45 to 65 degrees until the intervertebral foramina are clearly visualized. Most c-arms are limited in their ability to rotate obliquely to the side opposite the mobile base (the limit is typically 45 to 55 degrees). When performing cervical transforaminal injection on the side opposite the base unit, the limits of oblique angulation can be overcome by placing a foam wedge beneath the patient to angle them toward the side of the base unit, thereby gaining an additional degree of oblique angulation toward the opposite side. The limits of oblique angulation can also be overcome by inverting the c-arm so the x-ray source is above the patient and the image intensifier below; however, this results in a dramatic increase in radiation exposure to both the patient and the operator (see Fig. 2-5).

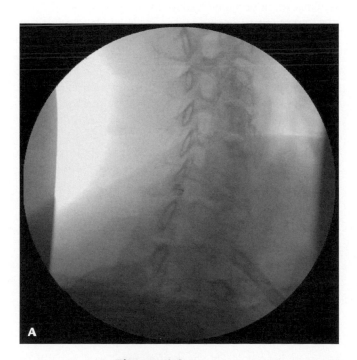
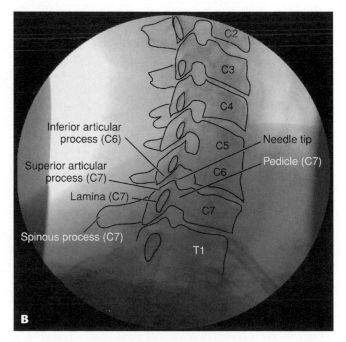

Figure 6-3.

Right oblique view of the cervical spine during right C6/C7 transforaminal injection. **A:** The needle is in proper position in the posterior aspect of the foramen for right C6/C7 transforaminal injection (C7 nerve root). Note that this patient has had a prior C5/C6 interbody fusion, and there is no discernible disc space between these two vertebrae. **B:** Labeled image.

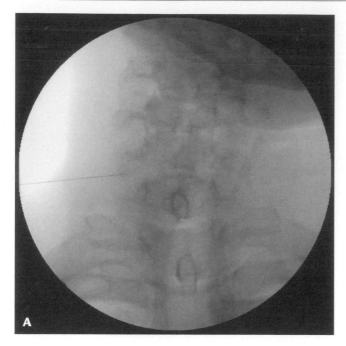
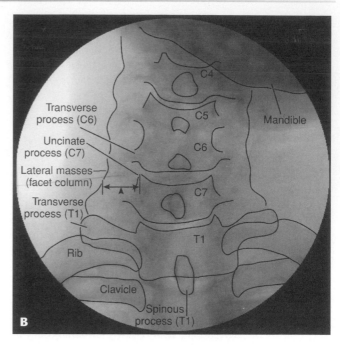

Figure 6-4.

Posterior-Anterior view of the cervical spine during C6/C7 transforaminal injection. **A:** The needle is in proper position within the right C6/C7 intervertebral foramen (C7 nerve root). Note that this patient has had a prior C5/C6 interbody fusion, and there is no discernible disc space between these two vertebrae. **B:** Labeled image.

advanced toward the posterior aspect of the intervertebral foramen midway between the superior and inferior limits of the foramen (see Fig. 6-3). Care is taken to be sure the needle tip remains superimposed on the bone of the facet column during advancement. In this way, the superior articular process of the facet just posterior to the foramen is first contacted, preventing needle advancement through the foramen and into the spinal canal. Once the needle contacts the facet, it is then walked anteriorly into the foramen and advanced no more than an additional 2 to 3 mm. The depth is then assessed by obtaining an image in the anterior-posterior (AP) plane (Fig. 6-4). To avoid direct trauma to the spinal cord and intrathecal injection, the needle should be advanced no further than halfway across the facet column. One to two milliliters of radiocontrast is then injected under "live" or real-time fluoroscopy to ensure the needle tip lies in close proximity to the nerve root without any intravascular or intrathecal spread (Fig. 6-5). The solution containing local anesthetic and/or steroid can then be injected safely (40 mg of triamcinolone acetonide or the equivalent and 0.5 to 1 mL of 1% lidocaine).

Complications

A firm grasp of the anatomy of adjacent vascular and neural structures is essential to avoid complications during cervical selective nerve root injection (see Fig. 6-1 *inset*). Direct intravascular injection into the vertebral artery may produce

generalized seizures when local anesthetic is used or cerebral ischemia when particulate steroid solutions are used. Direct injection of particulate steroid into a medullary artery supplying the spinal cord can lead to catastrophic spinal cord infarction. Needle positioning toward the posterior aspect of the foramen and advancing the needle in a plane parallel to the nerve root (rather than more anteriorly) reduces the risk of entering the vertebral artery. However, the use of radiographic contrast injected during "live" or "real-time" fluoroscopy (with or without digital subtraction) to visualize final needle position and detect any hint of intravascular injection is the only means to accurately verify that injectate is not injected within an artery (Fig. 6-6). Subarachnoid injection may also occur if the needle is advanced too medially and pierces the dural cuff as it extends laterally onto the exiting nerve root. Direct trauma to the exiting nerve root or the spinal cord itself may also occur.

Lumbar Transforaminal and Selective Nerve Root Injection

Anatomy

At typical lumbar levels, the ventral and dorsal roots of the spinal nerves descend in the vertebral canal to form the spinal nerves in their intervertebral foramina (Figs. 6-7 to 6-9). The foramen faces laterally. Its roof and floor are formed by the pedicles of consecutive vertebrae. Its posterior wall is formed largely by the superior articular process of the lower vertebra,

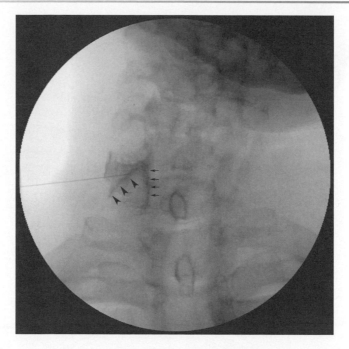

Figure 6-5.
Posterior-Anterior view of the cervical spine during C6/C7 transforaminal injection (after contrast injection). The needle is in final position within the right C6/C7 intervertebral foramen after injection of 1 mL of radiographic contrast medium (iohexol 180 mg per mL). Contrast outlines the exiting nerve root (*arrowheads*) and extends along the lateral aspect of the epidural space below the foramen (*small arrows*). (Reprinted from Rathmell JP, Aprill C, Bogduk N. Cervical transforaminal injection of steroids. *Anesthesiology* 2004:100:1,597, with permission.)

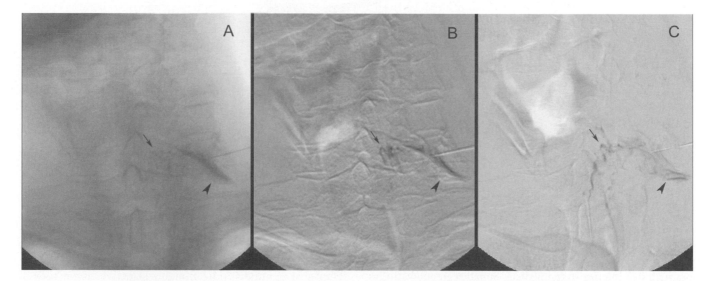

Figure 6-6.
Posterior-Anterior view of the cervical spine during C7/T1 transforaminal injection (digital subtraction sequence after contrast injection). An anteroposterior view of an angiogram obtained after injection of contrast medium, prior to planned transforaminal injection of corticosteroids. **A:** Image as seen on fluoroscopy. The needle lies in the left C7/T1 intervertebral foramen. Contrast medium outlines the exiting nerve root (*arrowhead*). The radicular artery appears as a thin thread passing medially from the site of injection (*small arrow*). **B:** Digital subtraction angiogram reveals the radicular artery extending medially more clearly (*small arrow*). **C:** Digital subtraction angiogram after pixel-shift reregistration reveals that the radicular artery (*small arrow*) extends to the midline to join the anterior spinal artery. (Reprinted from Rathmell JP, Aprill C, Bogduk N. Cervical transforaminal injection of steroids. *Anesthesiology.* 2004;100:1,597, with permission.)

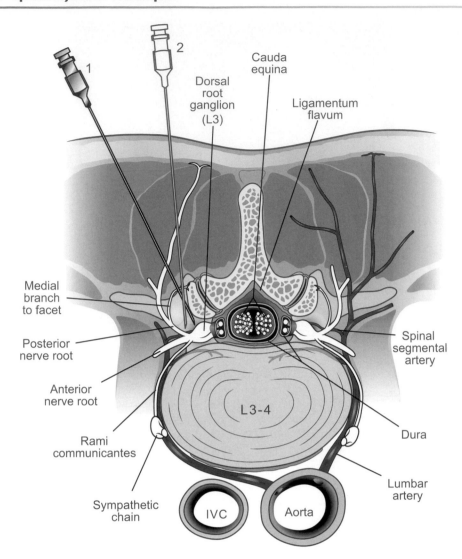

Figure 6-7.
Axial view of lumbar transforaminal and selective nerve root injection. The anatomy and proper needle position (axial view) for right (1) L3/L4 transforaminal injection and (2) L3 selective nerve root injection.

and in part by the inferior articular process of the upper vertebra and the capsule of the zygapophysial joint between the two articular processes. The anterior wall is formed by the vertebral body and the intervertebral disc. The spinal nerve, in its dural sleeve, lies in the anterior and superior portion of the foramen, just inferior to the pedicle. Spinal segmental arteries arise from the aorta and the iliac vessels and accompany the spinal nerve and its roots to the spinal cord. The location of the lumbar spinal segmental arteries is highly variable, but they can be present on either side as low as the L5/S1 interspace. The largest of the spinal segmental arteries is called the artery of Adamkiewicz, and typically enters the spinal canal from the left side between T9 and L1 (80% of individuals). However, the artery of Adamkiewicz can enter the spinal canal anywhere from T7 to L4. The artery typically enters the foramen along its ventral aspect within the superior half of the foramen. The final needle position during selective nerve root

or transforaminal injection lies in close proximity to both the exiting nerve root and the spinal segmental artery.

Patient Selection

The most common indication for selective nerve root or transforaminal injection is to place corticosteroid adjacent to an inflamed nerve root that is causing radicular symptoms. Nerve root inflammation may stem from an acutely herniated intervertebral disc causing nerve root irritation or other causes of nerve root impingement, such as isolated foraminal stenosis due to spondylitic spurring of the bony margins of the foramen. Selective nerve root injection with local anesthetic has also been employed diagnostically to determine which nerve root is causing symptoms when pathology exists at multiple vertebral levels. This information can prove helpful in planning surgical intervention.

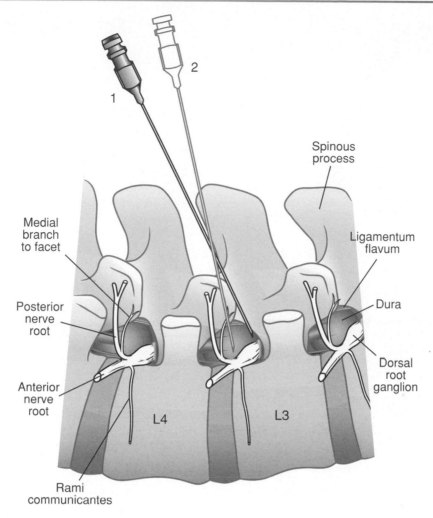

Figure 6-8.
Lateral view of lumbar transforaminal and selective nerve root injection. Anatomy and proper needle position (lateral view) for right (1) L3/L4 transforaminal injection and (2) L3 selective nerve root injection.

Positioning

The patient lies supine, facing directly forward (Fig. 6-10). The c-arm is rotated 20 to 30 degrees lateral oblique to allow direction of the needle toward the superolateral aspect of the intervertebral foramen (Fig. 6-11). A somewhat less oblique approach will result in a final needle position slightly lateral to the intervertebral foramen (see Figs. 6-7 and 6-8) and has been advocated by some practitioners as a means of limiting spread of the injectate to a single nerve root. However, even small volumes of injectate will often be seen to track along the exiting nerve root to enter the lateral epidural space.

Block Technique

A 22- or 25-gauge, 3.5-in spinal needle is sufficient in length for patients of average build, whereas a 5-in needle may be needed in obese patients. To avoid the exiting nerve root, the needle is advanced toward the superior aspect of the inter-

vertebral foramen, just inferior to the pedicle and inferolateral to the pars interarticularis (see Figs. 6-8 and 6-11). The needle tip can be advanced using a coaxial technique, and the tip first seated on the inferolateral margin of the pars interarticularis. This serves as an effective depth marker. Once this bony margin is contacted, the c-arm is rotated to a lateral view (Fig. 6-12), and the needle is slowly advanced toward the anterior and superior aspect of the foramen. If a paresthesia is reported by the patient at any time during needle advancement, the needle should be withdrawn slightly, and the position confirmed with radiographic contrast. With the needle in final position, 1 to 2 mL of radiographic contrast is injected under "live" or "real-time" fluoroscopy in the AP plane to ensure the needle tip lies in close proximity to the nerve root without any intravascular or intrathecal spread (Fig. 6-13). The injectate containing local anesthetic and/or steroid can then be injected safely. Obtaining a final lateral image will allow assessment of the extent of spread of the injectate (Fig. 6-14).

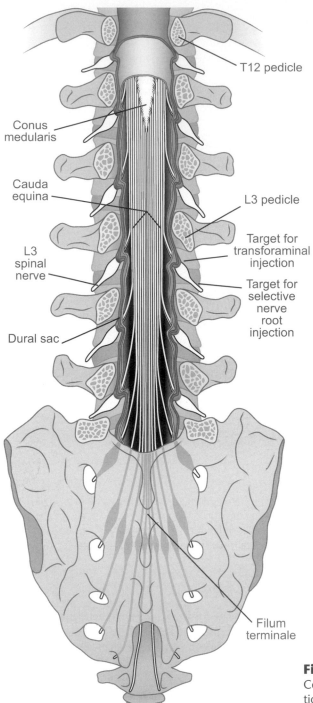

Conus
medularis

Cauda
equina

L3
spinal
nerve

Dural sac

T12 pedicle

L3 pedicle

Target for
transforaminal
injection

Target for
selective
nerve
root
injection

Filum
terminale

Figure 6-9.
Coronal view of lumbar transforaminal and selective nerve root injection. Anatomy and injection target points (coronal view) for L3/L4 transforaminal injection and L3 selective nerve root injection.

Complications

A firm grasp of the anatomy of adjacent vascular and neural structures is essential to avoid complications during lumbar selective nerve root and transforaminal injection (see Fig. 6-7). Direct injection of particulate steroid into a spinal segmental artery supplying the spinal cord can lead to catastrophic spinal cord infarction. Needle positioning toward the posterior aspect of the foramen reduces the risk of entering the spinal segmental artery. Particular care should be taken when performing transforaminal injection on the left between T9 and L1 because the artery of Adamkiewicz, the largest of the spinal segmental arteries, lies between these levels in the majority of individuals. The use of radiographic contrast injected during "live" or "real-time" fluoroscopy to visualize final needle position and detect any hint of intravascular injection is the only means to accurately verify that injectate is not injected within an artery. Subarachnoid

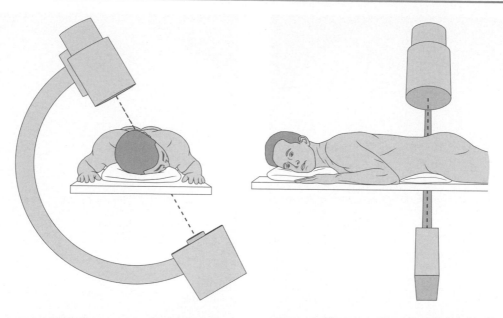

Figure 6-10.
Patient position for lumbar transforaminal and selective nerve root injection. The patient is positioned supine with c-arm axis rotated obliquely 20 to 30 degrees until the facet joint and pars interarticularis are clearly visualized.

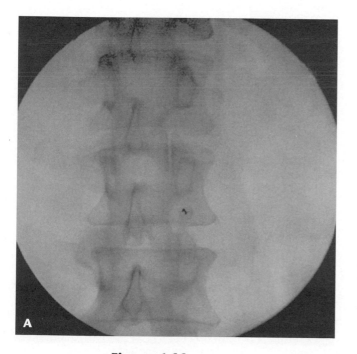

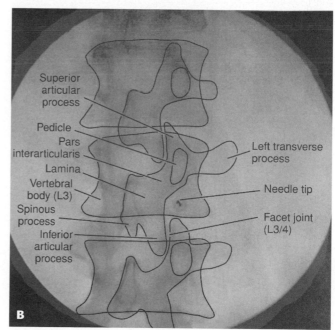

Figure 6-11.
Left oblique radiograph with needle in final position for right L3/L4 transforaminal injection. **A:** The needle tip lies directly inferior to the pedicle and inferolateral to the pars interarticularis. **B:** Labeled image.

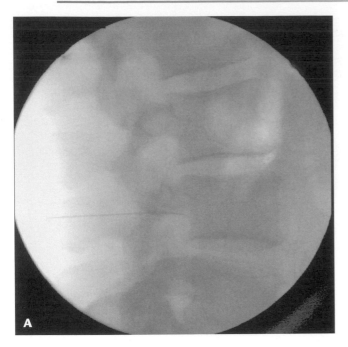

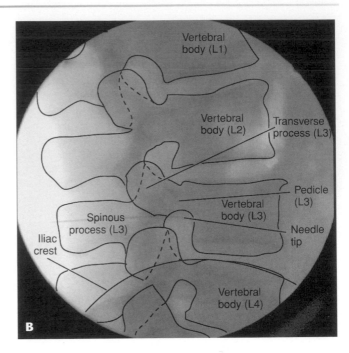

Figure 6-12.

Lateral radiograph with needle in final position for right L3/L4 transforaminal injection.
A: The needle tip lies directly inferior to the pedicle within the anterior and superior aspect
of the L3/L4 intervertebral foramen. **B:** Labeled image.

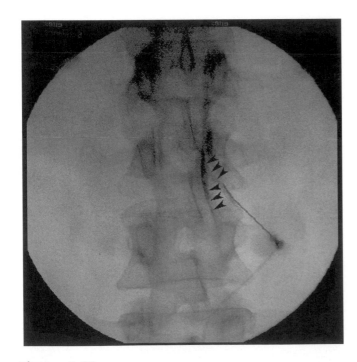

Figure 6-13.

Anterior-Posterior radiograph of the lumbar spine following lumbar transforaminal injection (after contrast injection). The needle
is in final position for left L3/L4 transforaminal injection following
injection of 1 mL of radiographic contrast. The needle tip lies
directly inferior to the pedicle and contrast extends to the left lateral epidural space beneath the pedicle (*upper group of arrowheads*). Contrast also extends along the left lateral aspect of the
epidural space to outline the L4 nerve root as it exits through the
left L4/L5 intervertebral foramen (*lower group of arrowheads*).

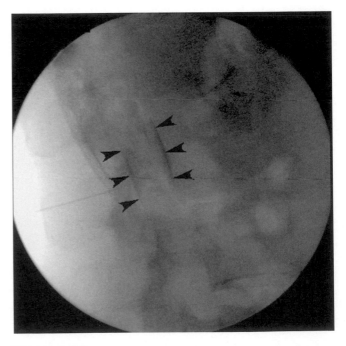

Figure 6-14.

Lateral radiograph of the lumbar spine following lumbar transforaminal injection. The needle is in final position for right
L3/L4 transforaminal injection following injection of 1 mL of
radiographic contrast. The contrast extends to the epidural
space, where it layers in both the anterior and posterior
epidural space forming two parallel lines characteristic of
epidural contrast placement (*arrowheads*).

injection may also occur if the needle is advanced too medially and pierces the dural cuff as it extends laterally onto the exiting nerve root. Direct trauma to the exiting nerve root or the spinal cord itself may also occur.

SUGGESTED READINGS

Baker R, Dreyfuss P, Mercer S et al. Cervical transforaminal injection of corticosteroids into a radicular artery: a possible mechanism for spinal cord injury. *Pain.* 2002;103:211–215.

Bogduk N. Diagnostic nerve blocks in chronic pain. *Best Pract Res Clin Anaesthesiol.* 2002;16:565–578.

Botwin K, Gruber R, Bouchlas C et al. Fluoroscopically guided lumbar transforaminal epidural steroid injections in degenerative lumbar stenosis: an outcome study. PG-898-905. *Am J Phys Med Rehabil.* 2002;81:898–905.

Bush K, Hillier S. Outcome of cervical radiculopathy treated with peri-radicular/epidural corticosteroid injections: a prospective study with independent clinical review. *Eur Spine J.* 1996;5:319–325.

Dooley J, McBroom R, Taguchi T et al. Nerve root infiltration in the diagnosis of radicular pain. *Spine.* 1988;13:79–83.

Furman MB, Giovanniello MT, O'Brien EM. Incidence of intravascular penetration in transforaminal cervical epidural steroid injections. *Spine.* 2003;28:21–25.

Furman MB, O'Brien EM. Is it really possible to do a selective nerve root block? *Pain.* 2000;85:526.

Gajraj NM. Selective nerve root blocks for low back pain and radiculopathy. *Reg Anesth Pain Med.* 2004;29:243–256.

Haueisen D, Smith B, Myers S et al. The diagnostic accuracy of spinal nerve injection studies. Their role in the evaluation of recurrent sciatica. *Clin Orthop.* 1985;198:179–183.

Herron L. Selective nerve root block in patient selection for lumbar surgery: surgical results. *J Spinal Disord.* 1989;2:75–79.

Hogan Q, Abram S. Neural blockade for diagnosis and prognosis. A review. *Anesthesiology.* 1997;86:216–241.

Houten JK, Errico TJ. Paraplegia after lumbosacral nerve root block: report of three cases. *Spine J.* 2002;2:70–75.

Karppinen J, Malmivaara A, Kurunlahti M et al. Periradicular infiltration for sciatica. a randomized controlled trial. *Spine.* 2001;26:1,059–1,067.

Lutz G, Vad V, Wisneski R. Fluoroscopic transforaminal lumbar epidural steroids: an outcome study. *Arch Phys Med Rehabil.* 1998;79:1,362–1,366.

North RB, Kidd DH, Zahurak M et al. Specificity of diagnostic nerve blocks: a prospective, randomized study of sciatica due to lumbosacral spine disease. *Pain.* 1996;65:77–85.

Pfirrmann C, Oberholzer P, Zanetti M et al. Selective nerve root blocks for the treatment of sciatica: evaluation of injection site and effectiveness—a study with patients and cadavers. *Radiology.* 2001;221:707–711.

Porter D, Valentine A, Bradford R. A retrospective study to assess the results of CT-directed peri-neural root infiltration in a cohort of 56 patients with low back pain and sciatica. *Br J Neurosurg.* 1999;13:290–293.

Rathmell JP, Aprill C, Bogduk N. Cervical transforaminal injection of steroids. *Anesthesiology.* 2004;100:1,595–1,600.

Renfrew DL, Moore TE, Kathol MH et al. Correct placement of epidural steroid injections: fluoroscopic guidance and contrast administration. *Am J Neuroradiol.* 1991;12:1,003–1,007.

Riew KD, Yin Y, Gilula L et al. The effect of nerve-root injections on the need for operative treatment of lumbar radicular pain: a prospective, randomized, controlled, double-blind study. *J Bone Joint Surg Am.* 2000;82:1,589–1,593.

Saal J. General principles of diagnostic testing as related to painful lumbar spine disorders: a critical appraisal of current diagnostic techniques. *Spine.* 2002;27:2,538–2,545.

Slipman CW, Lipetz JS, Jackson HB et al. Therapeutic selective nerve root block in the nonsurgical treatment of atraumatic cervical spondylotic radicular pain: a retrospective analysis with independent clinical review. *Arch Phys Med Rehabil.* 2000;81:741–746.

Stanley D, McLaren M, Euinton H et al. A prospective study of nerve root infiltration in the diagnosis of sciatica. A comparison with radiculography, computed tomography, and operative findings. *Spine.* 1990;16:540–543.

Vad V, Bhat A, Lutz G, Cammisa F. Transforaminal epidural steroid injections in lumbosacral radiculopathy: a prospective randomized study. *Spine.* 2002;27:11–16.

Vallee JN, Feydy A, Carlier RY et al. Chronic cervical radiculopathy: lateral approach periradicular corticosteroid injection. *Radiology.* 2001;218:886–892.

Windsor R, Pinzon E, Gore H. Complications of common selective spinal injections: prevention and management. *Am J Orthop.* 2000;29:759–770.

CHAPTER 7

Facet Injection: Intra-articular Injection, Medial Branch Block, and Radiofrequency Treatment

Overview

Intra-articular facet injection has been largely supplanted by radiofrequency treatment techniques for facet-related pain. Clinical experience and a limited number of published observational studies suggest that the intra-articular injection of local anesthetic and steroid leads to relief of facet-related pain that is limited in duration. In contrast, radiofrequency treatment is safe and modestly effective in producing longer-term pain relief in the same group of patients (see Facet Medial Branch Block and Radiofrequency Treatment section later in this chapter). Nonetheless, an understanding of facet-related pain syndromes and the methods for placing medication directly within the facet joint may still prove useful for those practitioners who are unable to provide radiofrequency treatment.

Osteoarthritis of the spine is ubiquitous and an inevitable part of aging. The degenerative cascade that leads to degeneration of the intervertebral discs causes progressive disc dehydration and loss of disc height. Typically starting in the third decade of life, disc degeneration leads to increased mobility of adjacent vertebrae and increased shear forces on the facet joints themselves. This can lead to a pattern of pain over the axis of the spine that increases with movement, particularly with flexion and extension, but produces little or no pain radiating toward the extremities. In the past, the only available treatment for those with debilitating facet-related pain was segmental fusion of the spine to completely arrest motion within the painful portion of the spine.

The majority of patients will have pain that is gradual in onset and can be localized only to a general region of the spinal axis (i.e., high or low cervical spine, high or low thoracic spine, or high or low lumbar spine). However, a subgroup of patients will present with sudden onset of pain, often associated with trauma in the form of sudden flexion or hyperextension of the spine in the affected region. Diagnostic studies are invariably unrevealing, either showing no abnormalities or facet arthropathy at multiple levels. In those with pain of sudden onset, it may be possible to isolate one or more facets that are causing the pain. It is in these instances with sudden onset of well-localized pain that intra-articular facet injection with local anesthetic and steroid can prove most beneficial.

Anatomy

The zygapophysial or "facet" joints are paired structures that lie posterolaterally on the bony vertebrae at the junction of the lamina and pedicle medially, and the base of the transverse process laterally. The facet joints are true joints, with opposing cartilaginous surfaces and a true synovial lining, and they are subject to the same inflammatory and degenerative processes that affect other synovial joints throughout the body. Two opposing articular surfaces comprise each facet joint. The facet joint articular processes are named for the vertebra to which they belong. Thus, each vertebra has a superior articular process and an inferior articular process. This nomenclature can be confusing because the superior articular process of a given vertebra actually forms the inferior portion of each facet joint. The paired facet joints, along with the vertebral bodies and intervertebral discs, form the three weight-bearing support columns that distribute the axial load on the vertebral column while allowing for movement in various planes.

The structure and location of the facet joints is distinct in the cervical, thoracic, and lumbar regions (Fig. 7-1). The cervical facet joints are oriented nearly parallel to the axial plane, where the atlas (C1) articulates with the occiput, and become gradually more steeply angulated in a cephalad-to-caudad direction at lower cervical levels. The orientation of the cervical facet joints in a plane close to the axial plane allows for a great degree of rotation of the neck, as well as flexion and extension. The thoracic facet joints become even more steeply angulated, approaching the frontal plane. At midthoracic levels, the inferior articular process of the vertebra forming the superior portion of each thoracic facet joint lies directly posterior to the superior articular process, forming the inferior portion of each joint. This allows for some degree of flexion and extension, but limited rotation of the spinal column in the thorax. The steeply angled cephalad-to-caudad orientation of the thoracic facets also makes intra-articular injection difficult or impossible. The lumbar facet joints are angled with a somewhat oblique orientation, allowing for flexion, extension, and rotation that is greater than that in the thorax but less than in the cervical region. The orientation of the facet joints and the optimal angle of needle insertion for intra-articular facet injection are illustrated in Figure 7-1.

The sensory innervation to the facet joints is predictable, and the sensory nerves are easily accessible from the back. The spinal nerve at each level exits the intervertebral foramen and divides into anterior and posterior primary rami. The anterior ramus contains the majority of sensory and motor fibers at each vertebral level. The posterior primary ramus, in turn, divides into a lateral branch that provides innervation to the paraspinous musculature and a small, variable sensory distribution to the skin overlying the spinous processes, whereas the medial branch courses over the base of the transverse process, where it joins with the superior articular process of the facet joint and courses along the articular process to supply sensation to the joint. Each facet joint receives sensory innervation from the medial branch nerve at the same vertebral level, as well as from a descending branch from the vertebral level above, thus two medial branch nerves must be blocked to anesthetize each facet joint (e.g., medial branch blocks at the base of the L4 and L5 transverse processes are needed to anesthetize the L4/L5 facet joint). The specific course of the medial branch nerves and cannula position for radiofrequency treatment at specific spinal levels is discussed in the following sections.

Patient Selection

Patients with facet-related pain are difficult to distinguish from those with other causes of axial spinal pain. Some patients will present with sudden onset of pain following a significant flexion-extension (whiplash) injury, but more common is an insidious onset over months to years. Patients with myofascial or discogenic pain and, in the low back, those with sacroiliac dysfunction present with similar symptoms. Nonetheless, certain features can be helpful in differentiating facet-related pain from other causes of spinal pain. The pain caused by facet arthropathy is most pronounced over the axis of the spine itself and is typically maximal directly in the region of the most affected joints. The pain tends to be exacerbated by movement, particularly extension of the spine, which forces the inflamed articular surfaces of the facet joints together. However, axial spinal pain at rest or worsening with forward flexion or rotation of the spine is also a common feature. The most important historical feature is a predominance of axial spinal pain; those patients who report that the predominance of their pain is in the extremities are more likely to have acute or chronic radicular pain than facet-related pain. The quality of the pain is typically deep and aching, and waxes and wanes with activity. Burning or stabbing qualities suggest neuropathic pain rather than facet arthropathy. Diagnostic studies are often unrevealing. Patients with significant facet-related pain may have unremarkable plain radiographs and/or imaging studies of the spine, or there may be facet arthropathy at multiple levels. Patient selection for facet injection or radiofrequency treatment is empiric, and relies on excluding other causes of pain and a pattern of pain that corresponds to facet-related pain.

The patterns of pain caused by abnormalities in specific facet joints has been established by injecting a mild irritant (usually hypertonic saline) into specific facet joints in healthy volunteers and then recording the pattern of pain produced. This information is shown in Figures 7-2 to 7-4 for the cervical, thoracic, and lumbar regions, respectively. The levels treated are chosen by correlating the patient's report of pain to these pain diagrams. Occasionally, a patient will present with evidence of facet arthropathy and a pattern of pain that corresponds to a single level, but this is uncommon. Most patients will have more diffuse pain that can only be narrowed to a specific region. Treatment should be directed to the joint or joints that most closely matches the pattern of referred pain that has been established for each joint and that typically requires treatment at more than one level.

Intra-articular Facet Injection Versus Radiofrequency Treatment

Choosing between intra-articular facet injection and diagnostic medial branch blocks followed by radiofrequency treatment is a frequent scenario. Limited outcome studies of intra-articular injection, particularly at the cervical level,

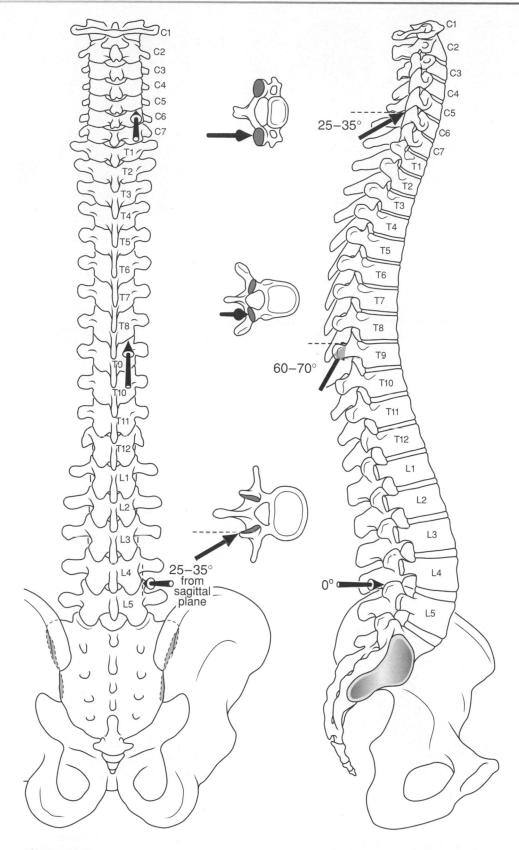

Figure 7-1.
Anatomy of the facet joints. The plane of orientation of the facet joints varies significantly among cervical, thoracic, and lumbar levels. The axis of the joints and the plane of entry for intra-articular injection are shown for typical cervical, thoracic, and lumbar facet joints.

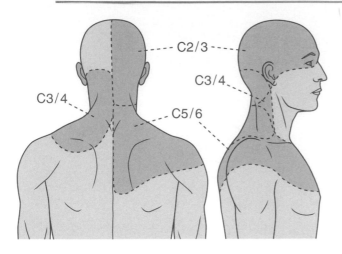

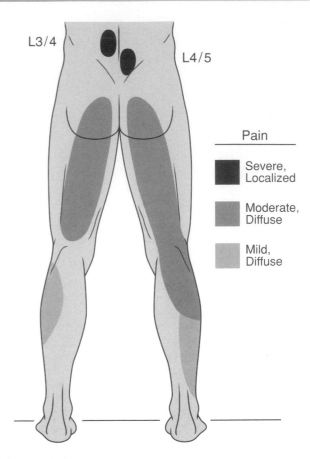

Figure 7-2.
Patterns of pain produced by cervical facet joints. Typical pain patterns produced by specific cervical facet joints are illustrated. Data are derived from intra-articular injection in healthy volunteers. (Data from Bogduk N, Marsland A. The cervical zygapophysial joints as a source of neck pain. *Spine.* 1988;13:615.)

Figure 7-4.
Patterns of pain produced by lumbar facet joints. Typical pain patterns produced by specific lumbar facet joints are illustrated. Data are derived from intra-articular injection in healthy volunteers. (Adapted from Boas RA. Facet joint injections. In: Stanton-Hicks MA, Boas RA, eds. *Chronic Low Back Pain.* New York: Raven Press; 1982:202, with permission.)

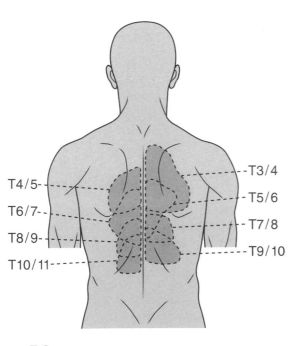

Figure 7-3.
Patterns of pain produced by thoracic facet joints. Typical pain patterns produced by specific thoracic facet joints are illustrated. Data are derived from intra-articular injection in healthy volunteers. (Adapted from Dreyfuss P, Tibiletti C, Dreyer S. Thoracic zygapophyseal joint pain patterns. *Spine.* 1994;19:809, with permission.)

have demonstrated only transient pain relief lasting from days to weeks in most patients. In contrast, in those patients who obtain significant pain relief from diagnostic blocks of the medial branch nerves to the facet, radiofrequency treatment can produce significant pain reduction that is somewhat longer lasting (typically 50% or more reduction in pain lasting at least 3 months after treatment). Based on this improved efficacy and a long track record of safety, more practitioners are beginning immediately with radiofrequency treatment rather than intra-articular injection. Intra-articular injection remains valuable in those patients who have recent onset of pain that is discrete in location and suggests involvement of a single facet joint. Intra-articular injection is also a reasonable alternative when the expertise or equipment for radiofrequency treatment is not available, but it will provide only transient symptomatic relief in those with facet-related pain who have failed conservative treatment.

Intra-articular Facet Injection

Cervical Intra-articular Facet Injection

Positioning

The patient lies prone, facing the table with a small headrest under the forehead to allow for air flow between the table and the patient's nose and mouth (Fig. 7-5). The c-arm is rotated 25 to 35 degrees caudally from the axial plane without any oblique angulation. This brings the axis of the x-rays in line with the axis of the facet joints and allows for good visualization of the joints (Fig. 7-6). Although the cervical facet joints can also be entered from a lateral approach with the patient lying on his or her side, advancing a needle using radiographic guidance in the anterior-posterior (AP) plane allows the operator to directly see the position of the spinal canal at all times and avoid medial needle deviation that could lead to spinal cord injury (Figs. 7-7 and 7-8).

Block Technique

The skin and subcutaneous tissues overlying the facet joint where the block is to be carried out are anesthetized with 1 to 2 mL of 1% lidocaine. The cervical level is easily identified by counting upward from the T1 level, where the vertebra is easily distinguished by the presence of a large transverse process that articulates with the first rib (see Fig. 7-6). A 22-gauge, 3.5-inch spinal needle is placed through the skin and advanced until it is seated in the tissues in a plane that is coaxial with the axis of the x-ray path (see Fig. 7-6). The needle is adjusted to remain coaxial and advanced toward the joint space using repeat images after every 2 to 4 mm of needle advancement. Once the surface of the joint space is contacted, a lateral radiograph is obtained (Fig. 7-9), and the needle is advanced just slightly to penetrate the posterior joint capsule. The needle should not be advanced into the joint between articular surfaces; this serves no purpose and is likely to abrade the articular surfaces and lead to worsened pain once the local anesthetic block subsides. Although intra-articular location of the needle tip can be confirmed with radiographic contrast, this is unnecessary if the needle location is correct in both AP and lateral planes. The facet joint itself holds only limited volume (typically <1 mL), and thus, placing contrast in the joint limits the ability to place local anesthetic and steroid within the joint. Once needle position has been confirmed, a solution containing steroid and local anesthetic is placed. A total dose of 80 mg of methylprednisolone acetate or the equivalent should be divided over all the joints to be injected, but more than 40 mg per joint is probably unnecessary. Using concentrated steroid (40 or 80 mg per mL) allows 1:1 mixture with local anesthetic (0.5% bupivacaine) to provide some immediate pain relief.

Thoracic Intra-articular Facet Injection

Positioning

Thoracic intra-articular facet injection is not commonly employed. The plane of the thoracic facet joints is steeply angled, nearing the frontal plane. Even with steep angulation of the c-arm, the joint space cannot be visualized directly, but rather it must be inferred from the position of adjacent structures. The patient is positioned prone with

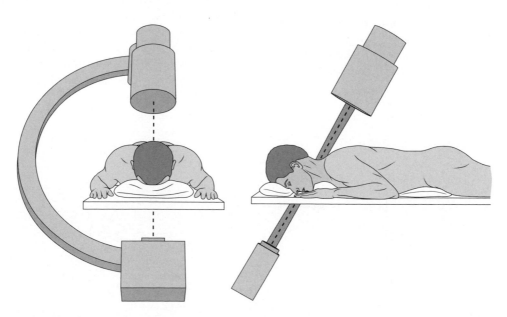

Figure 7-5.
Position for intra-articular cervical facet joint injection. The patient is placed prone with a small headrest under the forehead to allow for air flow between the table and the patient's nose and mouth. The c-arm is angled 25 to 35 degrees caudally from the axial plane.

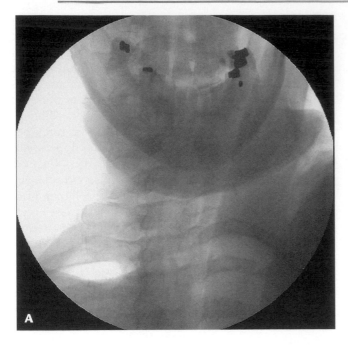

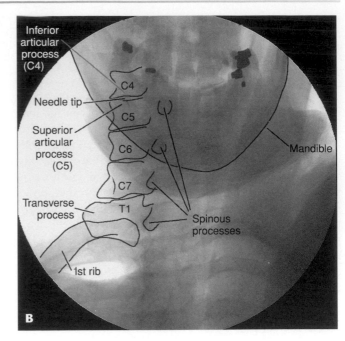

Figure 7-6.
Anterior-Posterior radiograph of the cervical spine during intra-articular cervical facet injection. **A:** A 22-gauge spinal needle is in position in the left C4/C5 facet joint. The needle tip is angled slightly to the left. **B:** Labeled image.

the head turned to one side. The c-arm is angled 50 to 60 degrees in a caudad direction from the axial plane (Fig. 7-10). The plane of the mid- and lower thoracic facet joints lies at an angle of 60 to 70 degrees from the axial plane, but further angulation of the c-arm is impractical without the image intensifier resting against the patient's back. This angle allows visualization of structures adjacent to the facet joint from which the position of the joint can be inferred (Fig. 7-11). The inferior articular process (superior aspect of the joint) lies posteriorly, directly over the superior articular process (inferior aspect of the joint). The needle tip is advanced toward the inferior aspect of the joint (Figs. 7-12 and 7-13).

Block Technique

The skin and subcutaneous tissues overlying the facet joint where the block is to be carried out are anesthetized with 1 to 2 mL of 1% lidocaine. The thoracic level is easily identified by counting upward from the T12 level, where the twelfth and lowest rib joins the T12 vertebra (see Fig. 7-11). A 22-gauge, 2-inch spinal needle (a 3-inch needle may be needed in obese patients) is placed through the skin and advanced until it is seated in the tissues in a plane that is coaxial with the axis of the x-ray path. The needle is adjusted to remain coaxial and advanced toward the inferior margin of the joint space (see Fig. 7-11). Because of the

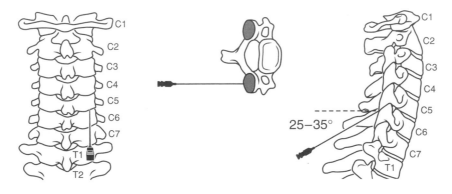

Figure 7-7.
Position and angle of needle entry for intra-articular cervical facet injection. A 22-gauge spinal needle is advanced in the sagittal plane overlying the facet joint with 25 to 35 degrees of caudad angulation from the axial plane.

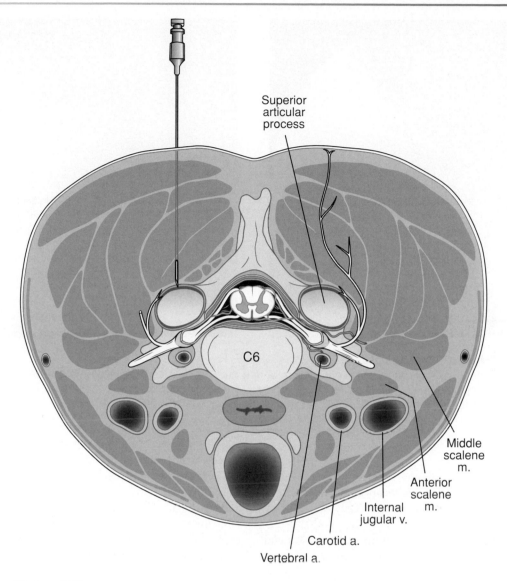

Figure 7-8.

Axial diagram of intra-articular cervical facet injection. The needle is advanced in the sagittal plane to enter the posterior aspect of the facet joint. Although the cervical facet joint can be entered from a lateral approach, using the posterior approach and radiographic guidance allows the operator to directly visualize the position of the spinal canal at all times. If the needle strays medially, the direction can be immediately corrected before dural puncture or injury to the spinal cord. When a needle is placed using a lateral approach, anterior deviation can also lead to penetration of the vertebral artery; the vertebral artery is protected by the facet column when a posterior approach is used.

joint's steep angle, the needle can be advanced only into the inferior- and posterior-most extent of the joint (see Fig. 7-13). Lateral radiography is difficult to interpret due to the overlying structures of the thorax. The facet joint itself holds only limited volume (typically <1 mL), and placing contrast in the joint limits the ability to place local anesthetic and steroid within the joint. Once the needle position has been confirmed, a solution containing steroid and local anesthetic is placed. A total dose of 80 mg of methylprednisolone acetate or the equivalent should be divided over all the joints to be injected, but more than 40 mg per joint is probably unnecessary. Using concentrated steroid (40 or

80 mg per mL) allows 1:1 mixture with local anesthetic (0.5% bupivacaine) to provide some immediate pain relief.

Lumbar Intra-articular Facet Injection

Positioning

The patient is positioned prone with the head turned to one side. The c-arm is angled obliquely 25 to 35 degrees from the sagittal plane and without caudal angulation (Fig. 7-14). This angle allows direct visualization of the facet joint (Figs. 7-15 to 7-17).

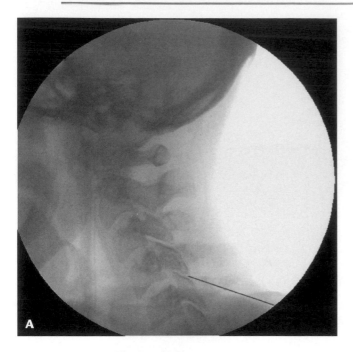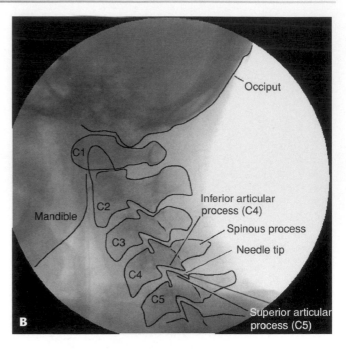

Figure 7-9.
Lateral radiograph of the cervical spine during intra-articular cervical facet injection. **A:** A 22-gauge spinal needle is in place in the posterior aspect of the C4/C5 facet joint. **B:** Labeled image.

Block Technique

The skin and subcutaneous tissues overlying the facet joint where the block is to be carried out are anesthetized with 1 to 2 mL of 1% lidocaine. The lumbar level is easily identified by counting upward from the sacrum (see Fig. 7-15). A 22-gauge, 3.5-inch spinal needle is placed through the skin and advanced until it is seated in the tissues in a plane that is coax-

ial with the axis of the x-ray path. The needle is adjusted to remain coaxial and advanced toward the joint space (see Fig. 7-15). The facet joint itself holds only limited volume (typically <1.5 mL), and placing contrast in the joint limits the ability to place local anesthetic and steroid within the joint. Nonetheless, intra-articular injection of contrast is commonly carried out at the lumbar levels. The articular space is z-shaped, with the superior recess extending slightly lateral to

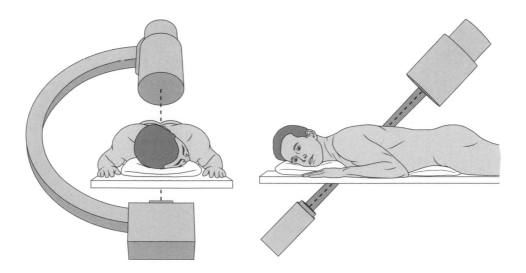

Figure 7-10.
Position for intra-articular thoracic facet joint injection. The patient is placed prone with the head turned to one side. The c-arm is angled 50 to 60 degrees caudally from the axial plane.

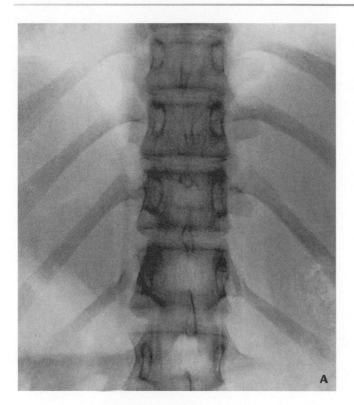
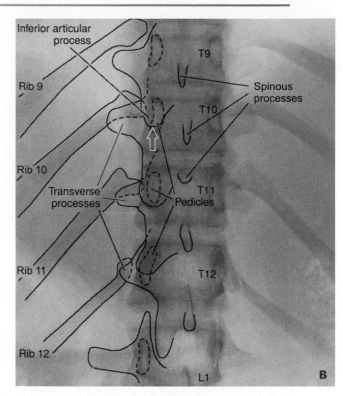

Figure 7-11.
Anterior-Posterior radiograph of the low thoracic spine. **A:** Because of their steep angle, the thoracic facet joints cannot be seen directly but must be inferred from the position of adjacent structures. The superior aspect of each joint (inferior articular process) lies posteriorly (*arrow*), directly over the inferior aspect of the joint (superior articular process). This position can be inferred by following the inferior margin of the lamina from the spinous process laterally. **B:** Labeled image.

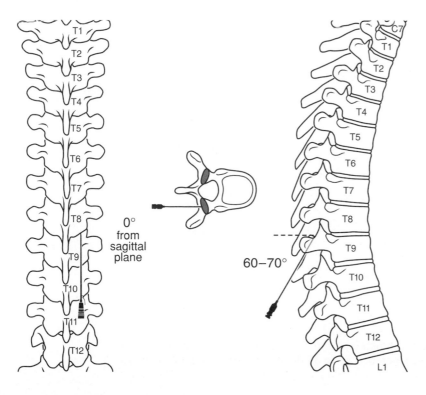

Figure 7-12.
Position and angle of needle entry for intra-articular thoracic facet injection. A 22-gauge spinal needle is advanced in the sagittal plane overlying the facet joint with 60 to 70 degrees of caudad angulation from the axial plane.

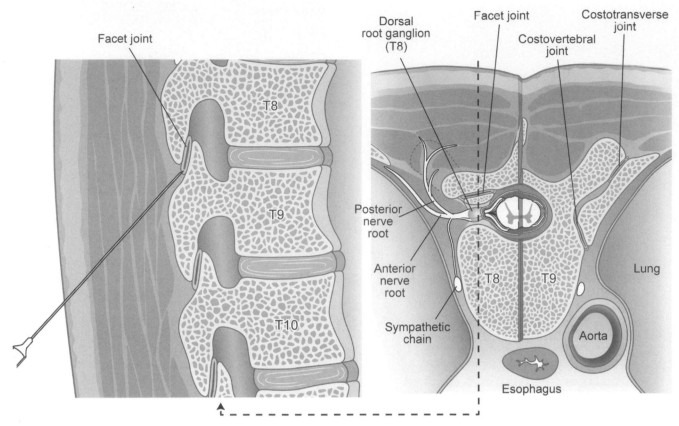

Figure 7-13.
Axial and sagittal diagrams of intra-articular thoracic facet injection. Axial panel (*right*): The needle is advanced in the sagittal plane to enter the posterior and inferior aspect of the facet joint. Sagittal panel (*left*): Because of the steep angle of the thoracic facet joints, the needle tip will only penetrate the posterior- and inferior-most aspect of the joint.

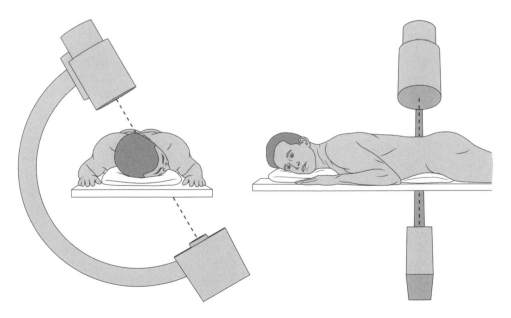

Figure 7-14.
Position for intra-articular lumbar facet joint injection. The patient is placed prone with the head turned to one side. The c-arm is angled 25 to 35 degrees from the sagittal plane parallel to the axial plane.

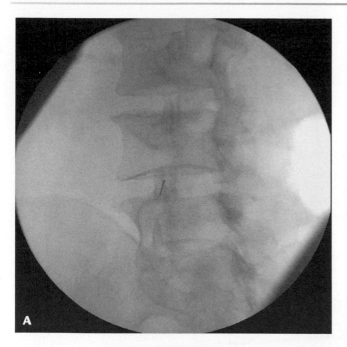
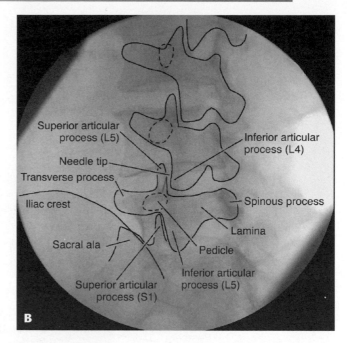

Figure 7-15.
Oblique radiograph of the lumbar spine during lumbar intra-articular facet injection.
A: The needle is in place in the left L4/L5 facet joint. The needle travels from inferior to
slightly superior. **B:** Labeled image.

the axis of the articular surfaces, and the inferior recess extending slightly medial to the axis of the articular surfaces (we do not routinely inject contrast). Once needle position has been confirmed, a solution containing steroid and local anesthetic is placed. A total dose of 80 mg of methylprednisolone acetate or the equivalent should be divided over all the joints to be injected, but more than 40 mg per joint is probably unnecessary. Using concentrated steroid (40 or 80 mg per mL) allows 1:1 mixture with local anesthetic (0.5% bupivacaine) to provide some immediate pain relief.

Complications of Intra-articular Facet Injection

Complications associated with intra-articular facet injection are uncommon. The most likely adverse effect is an exacerbation of pain. This is frequent when intra-articular cervical facet injection is carried out and the needle is advanced within the joint space. The joint space is narrow, and advancing the needle within the joint can abrade the articular surfaces, causing increased pain. This exacerbation

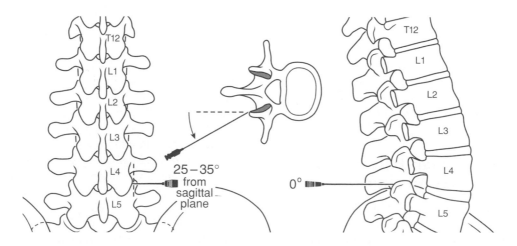

Figure 7-16.
Position and angle of needle entry for intra-articular lumbar facet injection. A 22-gauge
spinal needle is advanced in the axial plane overlying the facet joint with 25 to 35 degrees
of oblique angulation from the sagittal plane.

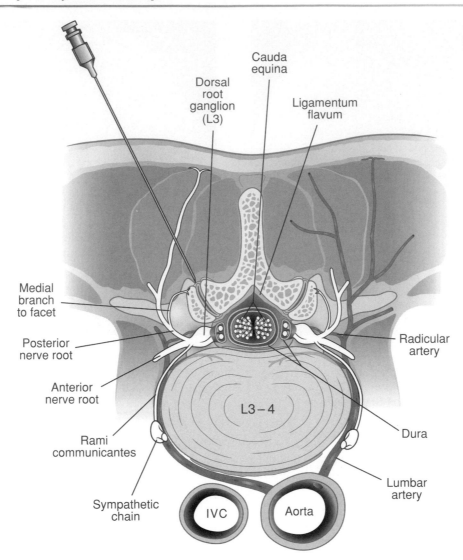

Figure 7-17.
Axial diagram of intra-articular lumbar facet injection. The axis of the facet joint lies 25 to 35 degrees from the sagittal plane. Note the innervation to the facet joint.

is usually self-limited. Infection can also occur, leading to abscess within the paraspinous musculature, but the incidence is exceedingly low. Bleeding complications have not been associated with intra-articular facet injection.

Facet Medial Branch Block and Radiofrequency Treatment

In those patients who receive only temporary relief from therapeutic intra-articular facet injections or who have pain that is more diffuse, requiring treatment at numerous levels, radiofrequency treatment can produce significant, enduring pain relief. Many investigators have pointed to the need for controlled diagnostic injections to determine who will respond to radiofrequency treatment. Despite the value of

placebo-controlled injections (i.e., comparative blocks with saline versus local anesthetic on different occasions), this is impractical in most clinical settings. Most practitioners rely on a single set of diagnostic local anesthetic blocks to the medial branch nerves at the levels of suspected pathology to determine who should receive radiofrequency treatment. Those who report significant pain relief, usually defined as 50% or greater pain reduction lasting the average duration of the local anesthetic, go on to radiofrequency treatment. Similarly transient pain relief with intra-articular injection of local anesthetic can also be used as a reasonable prognostic test before proceeding with radiofrequency treatment.

Conventional radiofrequency treatment produces a small area of tissue coagulation surrounding the active tip of an insulated cannula (Fig. 7-18). When the tip of the radiofrequency cannula is placed in close proximity to a

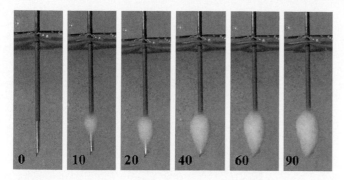

Figure 7-18.
Conventional radiofrequency lesion. A 10-cm SMK radiofrequency cannula with a 5-mm active tip is immersed in egg white and a lesion is carried out at 80°C for 90 seconds. The size of the lesion is maximal near the midportion of the active tip, with little coagulation at the tip of the needle. Thus, for optimal application of conventional radiofrequency treatment, the shaft of the needle's active tip must be placed adjacent to the target. The size of the lesion is near maximal by 60 seconds of treatment, changing little in size thereafter.

neural structure, the lesion encompasses the nerve causing denervation. The most commonly used cannulae for facet treatment are 22-gauge SMK (Sluijter-Mehta cannulae) and come in 5-, 10-, and 15-cm lengths with an active tip (non-insulated area where coagulation occurs) of 4, 5, or 10 mm; their placement is similar to placing a Quincke needle. For all but the most obese patients, the 10-cm cannulae with 5-mm active tips are used. In more recent years, pulsed radiofrequency treatment has come into frequent use. Pulsed radiofrequency produces voltage fluctuations at the tip of the cannula that are similar in magnitude to those produced during conventional radiofrequency treatment (40 to 50 V at 300 kHz). By applying the radiofrequency energy in intermittent pulses, the voltage fluctuations can be applied without heating of the tissue or resultant tissue coagulation. Pulsed radiofrequency has been shown to produce significant changes in gene expression within the dorsal horn of experimental animals, but evidence for the clinical efficacy of this approach is still lacking. The key concept when using conventional versus pulsed radiofrequency is to understand where the lesion or pulsed radiofrequency energy will occur relative to the active tip. The lesion produced by conventional radiofrequency is along the shaft of the needle surrounding the active tip (see Fig. 7-18). There is scant tissue destruction at the tip of the needle, thus the shaft of the active tip of the cannula must be placed along the course of the nerve. In contrast, the highest density of voltage change during pulsed radiofrequency emanates directly from the tip of the radiofrequency cannula, thus the tip of the needle should be directed along the course of the nerve to be treated. Techniques for both conventional and pulsed radiofrequency treatment will be discussed.

Cervical Medial Branch Block and Radiofrequency Treatment

Positioning

The medial branch nerves to the facets course across the articular pillar, midway between the superior and inferior articular processes (Fig. 7-19). The nerves can be anesthetized by placing a needle from a posterior approach (see Fig. 7-19) or a lateral approach (Figs. 7-20 and 7-21). For patients, the lateral approach is more comfortable because they can lie on one side rather than face down, and the needle must traverse less tissue en route to the target. However, when the needles are inserted from a lateral approach, they are directed toward the spinal cord. Even slight rotation of the neck can cause confusion among the left and right articular pillars and lead to needle entry into the spinal canal. For performing diagnostic medial branch blocks, either approach is adequate because the local anesthetic will be deposited in the same location with both approaches. For conventional radiofrequency treatment, the cannulae should be placed using a posterior approach because this will allow the entire length of the 5-mm active tip to align with the nerve on the articular pillar. For pulsed radiofrequency treatment, the cannulae can be placed from a lateral approach because the voltage fluctuations are maximal at the tip of the cannula.

Positioning for the Posterior Approach

The patient lies prone, facing the table with a small headrest under the forehead to allow for air flow between the table and the patient's nose and mouth (Fig. 7-22). The c-arm is rotated 25 to 35 degrees caudally from the axial plane without any oblique angulation. This brings the axis of the x-rays in line with the axis of the facet joints and allows for good visualization of the articular pillars (Fig. 7-23).

Positioning for the Lateral Approach

The patient lies in the lateral decubitus position with a pillow under the neck that minimizes lateral flexion of the neck to either side (Fig. 7-24). The c-arm is placed directly over the patient's neck without rotation or angulation. Care must be taken to ensure the left and right articular pillars are aligned directly over one another (Fig. 7-25). This is a point of great confusion among practitioners who are inexperienced with radiographic anatomy of the cervical spine. Even a small degree of rotation can place the left and right facet joints in significantly different locations on lateral radiographs. It is difficult to discern the left side from the right, and if a needle is advanced toward the contralateral facet target in error, the needle can easily pass into the spinal canal.

Block Technique: Diagnostic Medial Branch Blocks

The skin and subcutaneous tissues overlying the facet target where the block is to be carried out are anesthetized

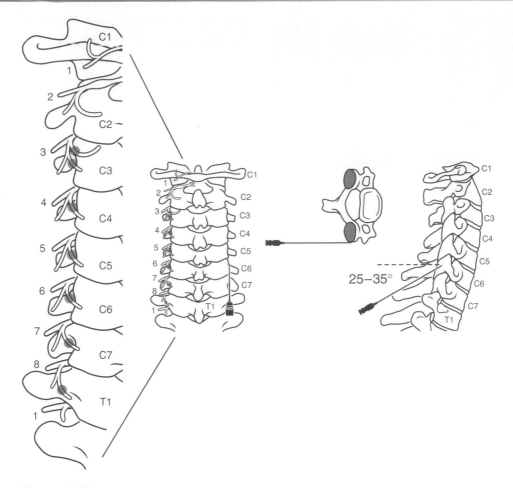

Figure 7-19.
Position and angle of needle entry for cervical medial branch blocks and radiofrequency treatment (posterior approach). A 22-gauge, 3.5-inch spinal needle (or 22-gauge, 10-cm SMK radiofrequency cannula with a 5-mm active tip) is advanced in a plane 25 to 35 degrees caudal to the axial plane toward the midpoint between superior and inferior articular processes of the facet to be treated. This point appears as an invagination or "waist," where the lateral margin of the facet column dips medially between articular surfaces. The target points for radiofrequency treatment are illustrated to the left. Note that treatment of the third occipital nerve requires that an additional cannula is placed toward the superior aspect of the C3 articular pillar overlying the C2/C3 facet joint.

with 1 mL of 1% lidocaine. The cervical level can be identified by counting upward from T1 (T1 is identified in the AP view by its large transverse process that articulates with the head of the first rib) or downward from C2 (C2 can be identified by its odontoid process in the AP view and its large spinous process in the lateral view). A 22-gauge, 3.5-inch spinal needle is placed through the skin and advanced until it is seated in the tissues in a plane that is coaxial with the axis of the x-ray path. The needle is adjusted to remain coaxial and advanced toward the facet target in the middle of the articular pillar, midway between superior and inferior articular surfaces of the vertebra. This appears as an invagination or "waist" on AP radiographs (see Fig. 7-23) and as a trapezoid on lateral radiographs (Fig. 7-26). From the posterior approach, the needle is gently seated on the lateral

margin of the facet column in the middle of the "waist"; from a lateral approach, the needle tip is seated in the middle of the trapezoid (see Figs. 7-19 to 7-21). Needle position is confirmed with AP and lateral radiographs (see Figs. 7-23 and 7-26). Once needle position has been confirmed, a small volume of local anesthetic is placed at each level and the needles are removed (0.5 mL of 2% lidocaine or 0.5% bupivacaine). The patient is instructed to assess his or her degree of pain relief in the hours immediately following the diagnostic blocks.

Block Technique: Radiofrequency Treatment

Radiofrequency cannulae are placed using a technique identical to that described for medial branch blocks. For

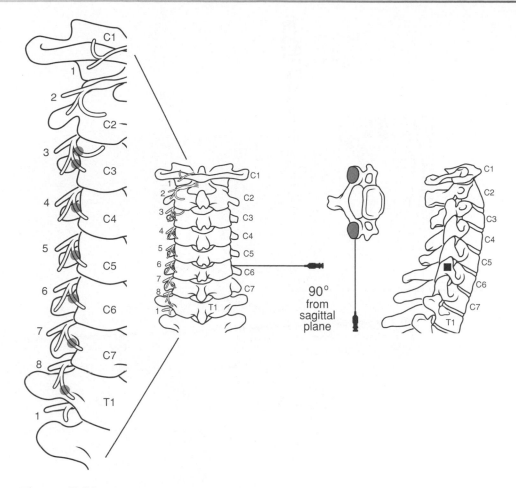

Figure 7-20.
Position and angle of needle entry for cervical medial branch blocks and radiofrequency treatment (lateral approach). A 22-gauge, 2-inch spinal needle (or 22-gauge, 5-cm SMK radiofrequency cannula with a 5-mm active tip) is advanced in the axial plane toward the midpoint between superior and inferior articular processes, and midway between the anterior and posterior borders of the facet column of the level to be treated. This point is in the center of the trapezoid that corresponds to the articular pillar of each vertebra when viewed from the side. The target points for radiofrequency treatment are illustrated to the left. Note that treatment of the third occipital nerve requires that an additional cannula is placed toward the superior aspect of the C3 articular pillar overlying the C2/C3 facet joint.

conventional radiofrequency treatment, 10-cm SMK cannulae with 5-mm active tips are used and placed from a posterior approach. Once the lateral margin of the facet column is contacted, the needle is walked laterally off the facet and advanced 2 to 3 mm to position the active tip along the course of the medial branch nerve (see Figs. 7-19 and 7-21). Proper testing for sensory-motor dissociation is conducted (the patient should report pain or tingling during stimulation at 50 Hz at less than 0.5 V, and have no motor stimulation to the affected myotome at 2 Hz at no less than three times the sensory threshold or 3 V). Thereafter, great care must be taken to prevent any movement of the cannulae. Each level is anesthetized with 0.5 mL of 2% lidocaine, and lesions are created at 80°C for 60 to 90 seconds.

For pulsed radiofrequency treatment, 5-cm cannulae with 5-mm active tips are inserted from a lateral approach. The tip is placed in the center of the trapezoid of the target facet, midway between articular surfaces, and midway between the anterior and posterior extent of the facet column (see Figs. 7-20 and 7-21). Proper testing for sensory thresholds is conducted (the patient should report pain or tingling during stimulation at 50 Hz at less than 0.5 V). Each level is then treated with pulsed radiofrequency adequate to maintain voltage fluctuations of 40 to 45 V for 120 seconds, without exceeding a tip temperature of 42°C. Local anesthesia is not needed for pulsed radiofrequency treatment, but it may be placed before the cannulae are removed.

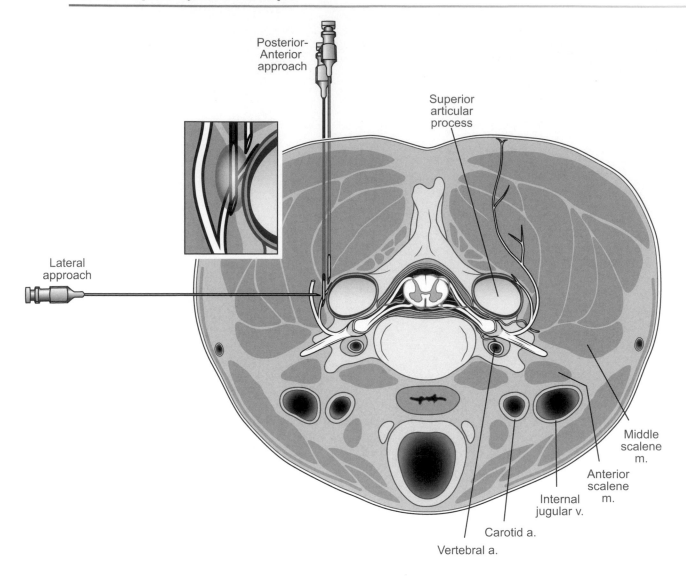

Figure 7-21.

Axial diagram of cervical medial branch nerve blocks and radiofrequency treatment. When needles are placed from a lateral approach, they are directed toward the spinal canal, and care must be taken to keep the needle tip over the bony facet target at all times as the needle is advanced. When a posterior approach is used, the needle is first seated on the lateral margin of the facet column. Local anesthetic can be placed without advancing the needle any further for diagnostic medial branch blocks. For conventional radiofrequency treatment, the cannulae must be walked off the lateral margin of the facet column and advanced 2 to 3 mm to place the active tip along the course of the medial branch nerve (*inset*).

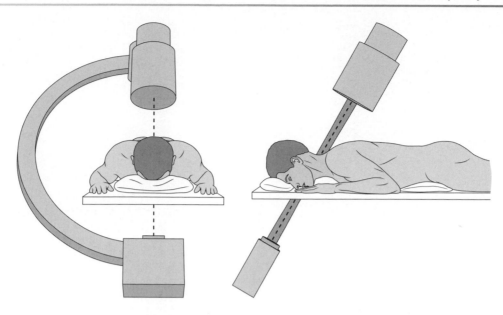

Figure 7-22.
Position for cervical medial branch blocks and radiofrequency treatment (posterior approach). The patient is placed prone with a small headrest under the forehead to allow for air flow between the table and the patient's nose and mouth. The c-arm is angled 25 to 35 degrees caudally from the axial plane.

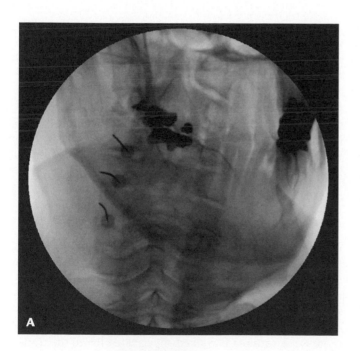

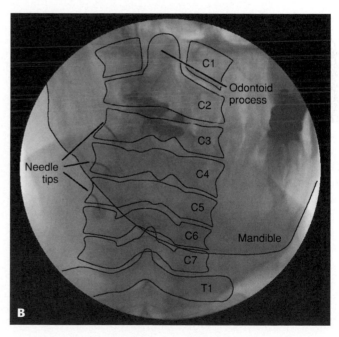

Figure 7-23.
Anterior-Posterior radiograph of the cervical spine during cervical medial branch block or radiofrequency treatment (posterior approach). **A:** Three radiofrequency cannulae are in place in the middle of the facet pillar at C3, C4, and C5 on the left. The caudad angulation of 25 to 35 degrees brings the facet joints into clear view and allows placement of the cannulae along the course of the medial branch nerves. **B:** Labeled image.

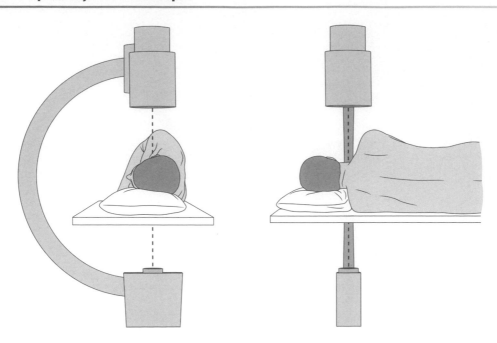

Figure 7-24.
Position for cervical medial branch blocks and radiofrequency treatment (lateral approach). The patient is placed on his or her side with a pillow under the head. The pillow should keep the cervical spine in alignment without lateral flexion to either side. The c-arm is placed directly over the patient's neck in the axial plane without angulation.

Thoracic Medial Branch Block and Radiofrequency Treatment

Positioning

The medial branch nerves typically cross the superolateral corners of the transverse processes and then pass medially and inferiorly across the posterior surfaces of the transverse processes (Figs. 7-27 and 7-28). At mid-thoracic levels (T5-T8), the curved course remains the same, but the inflection occurs at a point superior to the superolateral corner of the transverse process. The patient lies prone, with the head turned to one side (Fig. 7-29). The c-arm is positioned over the thoracic spine without angulation. The transverse processes of the thoracic vertebrae are best seen from this angle at both high (Fig. 7-30) and low (Fig. 7-31) thoracic levels.

Block Technique: Diagnostic Medial Branch Blocks

The skin and subcutaneous tissues overlying the facet target where the block is to be carried out are anesthetized with 1 mL of 1% lidocaine. The thoracic level can be identified by counting downward from T1 (T1 is identified in the AP view by its large transverse process that articulates with the head of the first rib) or upward from T12 (T12 articulates with the most inferior rib). A 22-gauge, 2-inch spinal needle is placed through the skin and advanced until it is seated in the tissues in a plane that is coaxial

with the axis of the x-ray path. The needle is adjusted to remain coaxial and advanced toward the superolateral margin of the transverse process (see Figs. 7-30 and 7-31) and is seated on the bony margin. Once the needle is in position, a small volume of local anesthetic is placed at each level, and the needles are removed (0.5 mL of 2% lidocaine or 0.5% bupivacaine). The patient is instructed to assess his or her degree of pain relief in the hours immediately following the diagnostic blocks.

Block Technique: Radiofrequency Treatment

Radiofrequency cannulae are placed using a technique identical to that described for medial branch blocks. For conventional radiofrequency treatment, 10-cm SMK cannulae with 5-mm active tips are used (5-cm cannulae are sufficient in length in all but obese patients). Once the needle is seated against the superior margin of the transverse process the cannula is walked superolaterally off the transverse process and advanced 2 to 3 mm to position the active tip along the course of the medial branch nerve (Figs. 7-28 and 7-32). Proper testing for sensory-motor dissociation is conducted (the patient should report pain or tingling during stimulation at 50 Hz at less than 0.5 V, and have no motor stimulation to the affected myotome of the chest wall at 2 Hz at no less than three times the sensory threshold or 3 V). Thereafter, great care must be taken to prevent any movement of the cannulae. Each level is

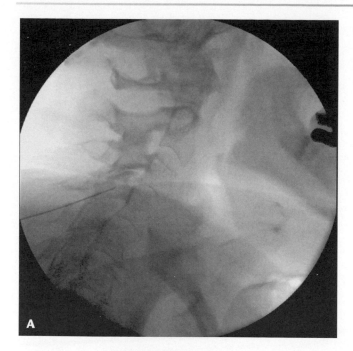
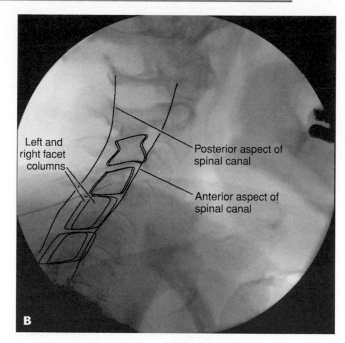

Figure 7-25.
Lateral radiograph of the cervical spine during cervical medial branch block (posterior approach) demonstrating poor alignment of the left and right facet columns. **A:** A single needle is seated in the middle of the articular pillar C4, midway between superior and inferior articular processes and midway between the anterior and posterior borders of the facet column (in the middle of the trapezoid). When needles are placed from a lateral approach, great care must be taken to align the left and right facet columns so that they are superimposed. Even small degrees of rotation place the left and right facets in different locations, as seen in the inferior part of the image, where the left and right C6 facet pillars are not aligned. It is difficult to distinguish the left from the right facet on a lateral radiograph, and if they are not superimposed, there is danger that a needle advanced from a lateral approach could be directed in error toward the contralateral facet and enter the spinal canal. **B:** Labeled image.

anesthetized with 0.5 mL of 2% lidocaine, and lesions are created at 80°C for 60 to 90 seconds. Cannula placement for thoracic pulsed radiofrequency treatment is carried out in the same manner.

Lumbar Medial Branch Block and Radiofrequency Treatment

Positioning

The medial branch nerves to the lumbar facets course over the base of the transverse process, where they join with the superior articular processes (Figs. 7-33 and 7-34). The medial branch nerve lies in the groove between the transverse process and the superior articular process, which slopes inferolaterally. The patient lies prone, with the head turned to one side (Fig. 7-35). A pillow is placed under the lower abdomen in an effort to tilt the pelvis backward and swing the iliac crests posteriorly away from the lumbosacral junction. The c-arm is positioned over the lumbar spine with 25 to 35 degrees of oblique angulation so the

facet joints, as well as the junction between the transverse process and the superior articular process, are clearly seen (Fig. 7-36). For medial branch blocks, the needle can be advanced in the axial plane without caudal angulation (see Fig. 7-33). However, for radiofrequency treatment, the c-arm should be angled 25 to 30 degrees caudal to the axial plane so the active tip of the radiofrequency cannulae will be parallel to the medial branch nerve within the groove between the transverse process and the superior articular process as it slopes inferomedially (see Fig. 7-33).

Block Technique: Diagnostic Medial Branch Blocks

The skin and subcutaneous tissues overlying the facet target where the block is to be carried out are anesthetized with 1 mL of 1% lidocaine. The lumbar level can be identified by counting upward from the sacrum. A 22-gauge, 3.5-inch spinal needle is placed through the skin and advanced until it is seated in the tissues in a plane that is coaxial with the axis of the x-ray path. The needle is adjusted to remain coaxial and advanced toward the base of the transverse

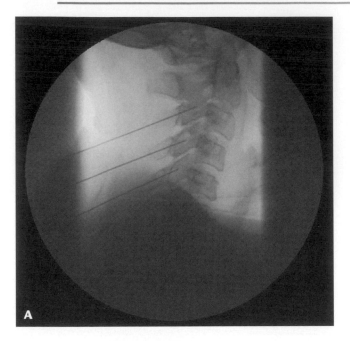
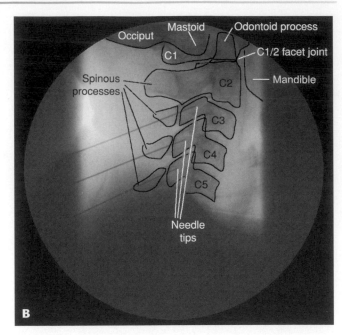

Figure 7-26.
Lateral radiograph of the cervical spine during cervical medial branch block or radiofrequency treatment (posterior approach). **A:** Three radiofrequency cannulae are in place in the middle of the facet pillar at C3, C4, and C5 on the left. The caudad angulation of 25 to 35 degrees allows placement of the cannulae along the course of the medial branch nerves, parallel to the articular surfaces. **B:** Labeled image.

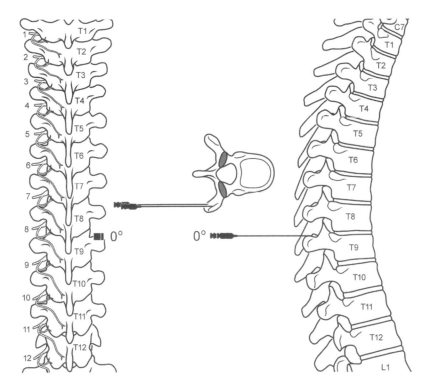

Figure 7-27.
Position and angle of needle entry thoracic medial branch blocks and radiofrequency treatment. A 22-gauge, 2-inch spinal needle (or 22-gauge, 5-cm SMK radiofrequency cannula with a 5-mm active tip) is advanced in the axial plane toward the superolateral margin of the transverse process. The target points for radiofrequency treatment are illustrated to the left.

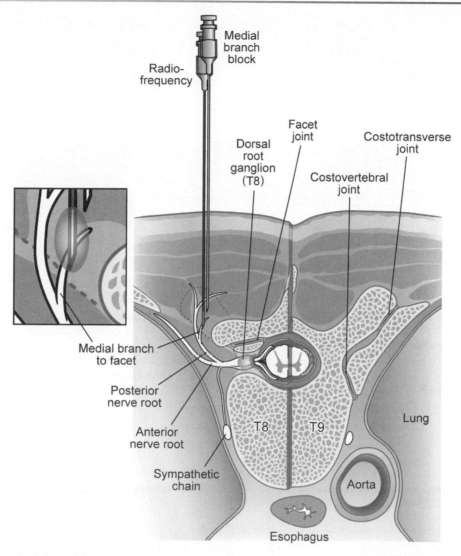

Figure 7-28.
Axial diagram of thoracic medial branch nerve blocks and radiofrequency treatment. A 22-gauge, 2-inch spinal needle (or 22-gauge, 5-cm SMK radiofrequency cannula with a 5-mm active tip) is advanced in the axial plane toward the superolateral margin of the transverse process. For conventional radiofrequency treatment, the cannulae must be walked off the superior margin of the transverse process and advanced 2 to 3 mm to place the active tip along the course of the medial branch nerve *(inset)*.

process, where it joins the superior articular process (see Figs. 7-33 to 7-36) and is seated on the bony margin. Once the needle is in position, a small volume of local anesthetic is placed at each level, and the needles are removed (0.5 mL of 2% lidocaine or 0.5% bupivacaine). The patient is instructed to assess his or her degree of pain relief in the hours immediately following the diagnostic blocks.

Block Technique: Radiofrequency Treatment

Radiofrequency cannulae are placed using a technique identical to that described for medial branch blocks; however, the c-arm is angled 25 to 30 degrees caudal to the

axial plane so the active tip of the radiofrequency cannulae will be parallel to the medial branch. For conventional radiofrequency treatment, 10-cm SMK cannulas with 5-mm active tips are used. Once the needle is seated against the superior margin of the transverse process, where it joins the superior articular process of the facet, the cannula is walked off the superior margin of the transverse process and advanced 2 to 3 mm to position the active tip along the course of the medial branch nerve (Figs. 7-33, 7-34, and 7-36 to 7-38). Proper testing for sensory-motor dissociation is conducted (the patient should report pain or tingling during stimulation at 50 Hz at less than 0.5 V, and have no motor stimulation to the affected myotome of the

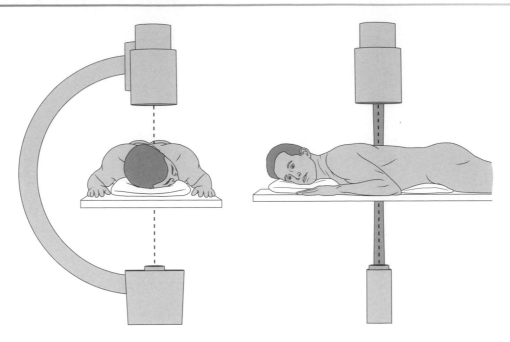

Figure 7-29.
Position for thoracic medial branch blocks and radiofrequency treatment. The patient is placed prone with the head turned to one side. The c-arm is positioned over the thoracic spine in a direct anterior-posterior plane without angulation.

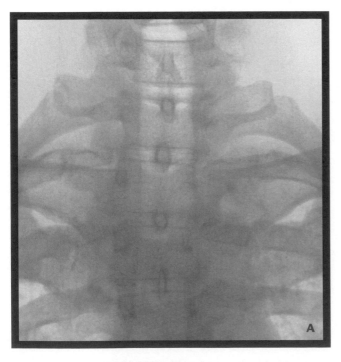
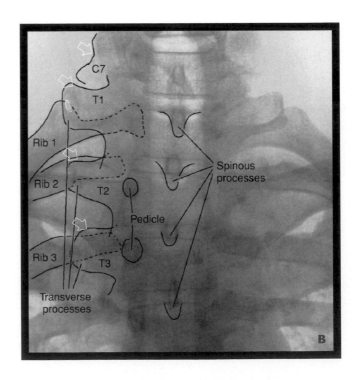

Figure 7-30.
Anterior-Posterior radiograph of the high thoracic spine. **A:** The transverse processes are prominent at high thoracic levels. The base of the transverse process joins the superior articular process just superolateral to the pedicle. **B:** Labeled image. The arrows indicate the targets for medial branch nerve blocks or radiofrequency treatment at the C7 to T3 levels on the left.

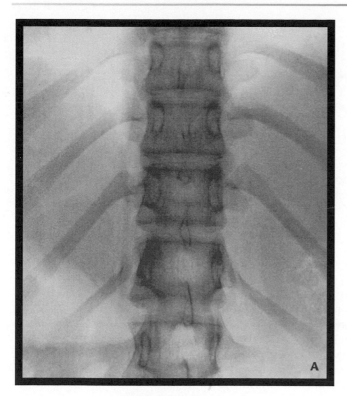 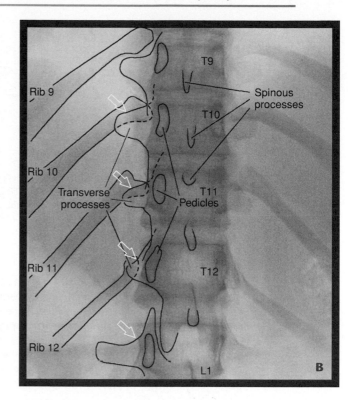

Figure 7-31.
Anterior-Posterior radiograph of the low thoracic spine. **A:** The transverse processes are less prominent at low thoracic levels, and often difficult to see at all at T12. The base of the transverse process joins the superior articular process just superolateral to the pedicle, and the pedicle is used as a landmark to locate the target for injection. **B:** Labeled image. The arrows indicate the targets for medial branch nerve blocks or radiofrequency treatment at T10 to L1 levels on the left.

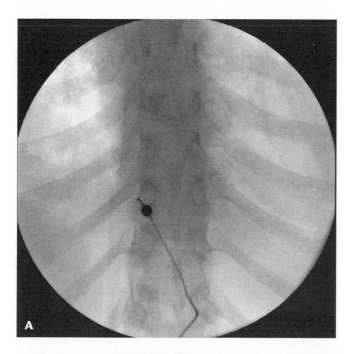 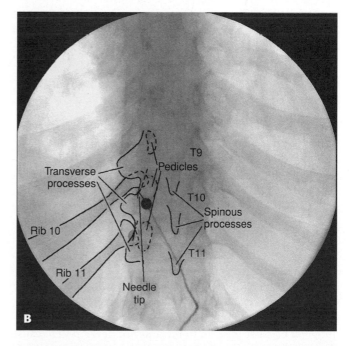

Figure 7-32.
Anterior-Posterior radiograph of the thoracic spine during radiofrequency treatment of the thoracic facets. **A:** A single radiofrequency cannulae is in place along the superolateral margin of the left T10 transverse process, where it joins the superior articular process. **B:** Labeled image.

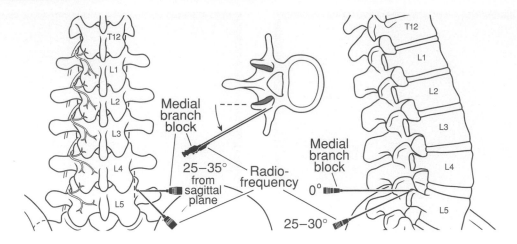

Figure 7-33.
Position and angle of needle entry for lumbar medial branch blocks and radiofrequency treatment. A 22-gauge, 3.5-inch spinal needle (or 22-gauge, 10-cm SMK radiofrequency cannula with a 5-mm active tip) is advanced toward the base of the transverse process, where it joins with the superior articular process. Cannulae placement for conventional radiofrequency treatment should be carried out with 25 to 30 degrees of caudal angulation of the c-arm to bring the axis of the active tip parallel to the course of the medial branch nerve in the groove between the transverse process and the superior articular process. The target points for radiofrequency treatment are illustrated to the left.

lower extremity at 2 Hz at no less than three times the sensory threshold or 3 V). Thereafter, great care must be taken to prevent any movement of the cannulae. Each level is anesthetized with 0.5 mL of 2% lidocaine, and lesions are created at 80°C for 60 to 90 seconds. Cannula placement for lumbar pulsed radiofrequency treatment is carried out in the same manner.

Complications of Medial Branch Block and Radiofrequency Treatment

Complications associated with diagnostic medial branch nerve blocks are uncommon and similar to those following intra-articular facet injection. Unlike intra-articular injection, it is unusual for medial branch blocks to cause an exacerbation of pain. Patients should be warned to expect mild pain at the injection site lasting a day or two after the procedure. Radiofrequency treatment of the facets is also associated with few complications. Although conventional radiofrequency produces actual tissue destruction, injury to the spinal nerves is uncommon. This is likely due to the physiologic testing before each lesion. As long as proper sensory and motor testing are carried out before each lesion is created, there is little chance that the active tip of the cannula will be close enough to the anterior nerve root to cause injury. Exacerbation of pain following conventional radiofrequency treatment is common, and patients should be instructed to expect an increase in pain similar in character to their usual pain that will last from several days to a

week or more. A smaller group of patients will report uncomfortable dysesthesia, usually in the form of a sunburned feeling of the skin overlying the spinous processes at the level of treatment often accompanied by allodynia (pain to light touch in the area). This adverse effect is more common following cervical radiofrequency treatment and usually subsides over several weeks. These dysesthesia likely stem from partial denervation of the lateral branch of the posterior primary ramus, which supplies a variable region of cutaneous innervation overlying the spinous processes. Likewise, some patients will report a small patch of complete sensory loss in this same region. Injury to the spinal nerve root with new-onset radicular pain with or without radiculopathy (nerve root dysfunction in the distribution of the spinal nerve in the form of sensory or motor loss) has been reported following radiofrequency treatment, but it should be rare when physiologic testing is employed. Pulsed radiofrequency treatment does not produce tissue destruction; thus, it is not surprising that most patients will have no worsening of their pain following treatment or a transient, mild exacerbation that is short lived. Painful dysesthesia and other consequences of nerve injury do not occur with pulsed radiofrequency treatment. It is precisely because of this lack of neural destruction and associated adverse effects that pulsed radiofrequency treatment has become so popular among practitioners. If controlled trials emerge to support the efficacy of pulsed radiofrequency treatment, it will rapidly replace conventional radiofrequency.

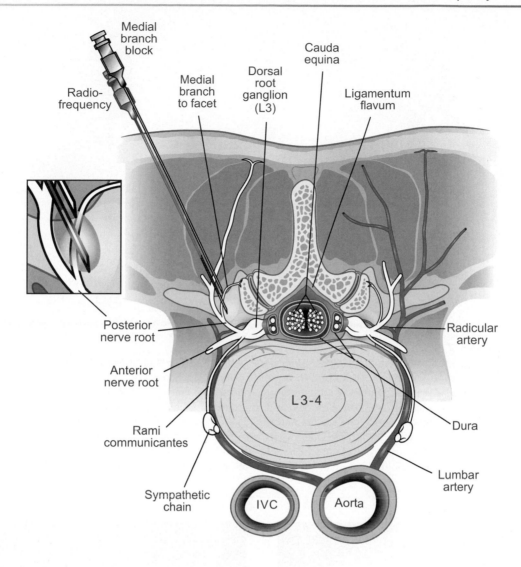

Figure 7-34.
Axial diagram of lumbar medial branch nerve blocks and radiofrequency treatment. A 22-gauge, 3.5-inch spinal needle (or 22-gauge, 10-cm SMK radiofrequency cannula with a 5-mm active tip) is advanced toward the base of the transverse process, where it joins with the superior articular process. Cannulae placement for conventional radiofrequency treatment should be carried out with 25 to 30 degrees of caudal angulation of the c-arm to bring the axis of the active tip parallel to the course of the medial branch nerve in the groove between the transverse process and the superior articular process. For conventional radiofrequency treatment, the cannulae must be walked off the superior margin of the transverse process and advanced 2 to 3 mm to place the active tip along the course of the medial branch nerve (*inset*).

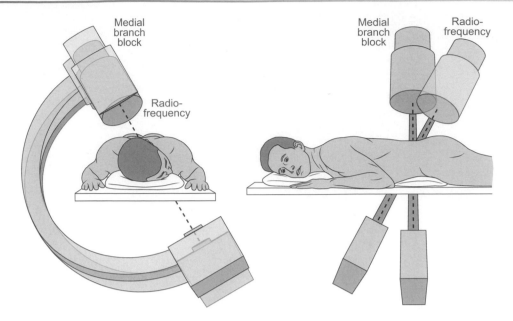

Figure 7-35.
Position for lumbar medial branch blocks and radiofrequency treatment. The patient is placed prone with the head turned to one side. The c-arm is positioned over the lumbar spine with 25 to 35 degrees of oblique angulation so the facet joints themselves and the junction between the transverse process and the superior articular process are clearly seen. For medial branch blocks, the needle can be advanced in the axial plane without caudal angulation. However, for radiofrequency treatment, the c-arm should be angled 25 to 30 degrees caudal to the axial plane so the active tip of the radiofrequency cannulae will be parallel to the medial branch nerve in the groove between the transverse process and the superior articular process.

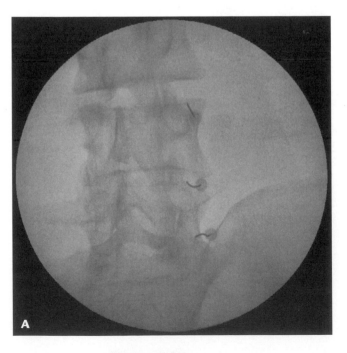

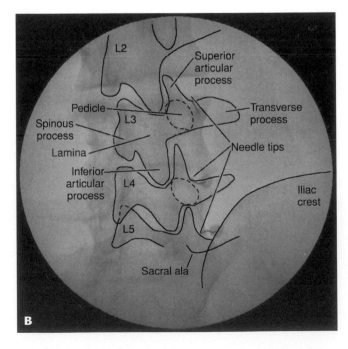

Figure 7-36.
Oblique radiograph of the lumbar spine during lumbar radiofrequency treatment of the lumbar facet joints. **A:** Three radiofrequency cannulae are in place at the base of the transverse processes and superior articular processes at the L3, L4, and L5 levels on the right. **B:** Labeled image.

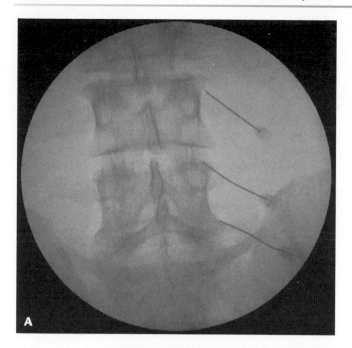
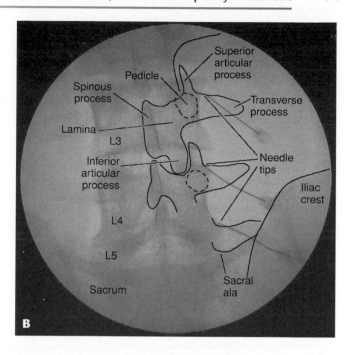

Figure 7-37.
Anterior-Posterior radiograph of the lumbar spine during lumbar radiofrequency treatment of the lumbar facet joints. **A:** Three radiofrequency cannulae are in place at the base of the transverse processes and superior articular processes at the L3, L4, and L5 levels on the right. Note the angle of the entering cannulae. **B:** Labeled image.

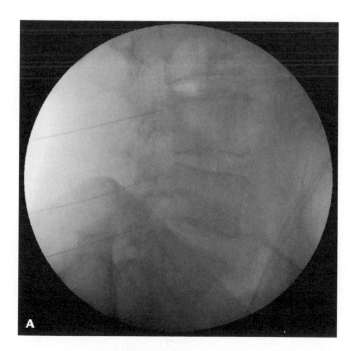
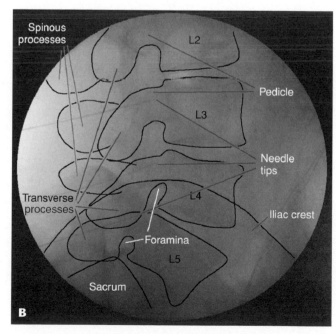

Figure 7-38.
Lateral radiograph of the lumbar spine during lumbar radiofrequency treatment of the lumbar facet joints. **A:** Three radiofrequency cannulae are in place at the base of the transverse processes and superior articular processes at the L3, L4, and L5 levels on the right. Note the angle of the entering cannulae and their distance from the intervertebral foramina. **B:** Labeled image.

SUGGESTED READINGS

Bogduk N, Holmes S. Controlled zygapophysial joint blocks: the travesty of cost-effectiveness. *Pain Med.* 2000;1:24–34.

Bogduk N, Marsland A. The cervical zygapophysial joints as a source of neck pain. *Spine.* 1988;13:610–617.

Chua WH, Bogduk N. The surgical anatomy of thoracic facet denervation. *Acta Neurochir (Wien).* 1995;136:140–144.

Coskun DJ, Gilchrist J, Dupuy D. Lumbosacral radiculopathy following radiofrequency ablation therapy. *Muscle Nerve.* 2003;28:754–756.

Dreyer SJ, Dreyfuss PH. Low back pain and the zygapophysial (facet) joints. *Arch Phys Med Rehabil.* 1996;77:290–300.

Dreyfuss P, Baker R, Leclaire R et al. Radiofrequency facet joint denervation in the treatment of low back pain: a placebo-controlled clinical trial to assess efficacy. *Spine.* 2002;27:556–557.

Govind J, King W, Bailey B et al. Radiofrequency neurotomy for the treatment of third occipital headache. *J Neurol Neurosurg Psychiatry.* 2003;74:88–93.

Lord SM, Barnsley L, Wallis BJ et al. Percutaneous radio-frequency neurotomy for chronic cervical zygapophyseal-joint pain. *N Engl J Med.* 1996;335:1,721–1,726.

Mikeladze G, Espinal R, Finnegan R et al. Pulsed radiofrequency application in treatment of chronic zygapophyseal joint pain. *Spine J.* 2003;3:360–362.

Niemisto L, Kalso E, Malmivaara A et al. Radiofrequency denervation for neck and back pain: a systematic review within the framework of the Cochrane Collaboration Back Review Group. *Spine.* 2003;28: 1,877–1,888.

Slipman CW, Bhat AL, Gilchrist RV et al. A critical review of the evidence for the use of zygapophysial injections and radiofrequency denervation in the treatment of low back pain. *Spine J.* 2003;3:310–316.

Sacroiliac Joint Injection

Overview

Pain arising from the sacroiliac (SI) joints is common and difficult to distinguish from other causes of pain in the area of the lumbosacral junction. SI joint dysfunction typically presents with localized pain in the lower back or upper buttock overlying the SI joint. Pain may be referred to the posterior thigh, but pain extending below the knee is unusual. In most cases, the etiology is unclear, and the onset is gradual over months to years. Trauma, infection, and tumor are uncommon causes of SI joint pain. The inflammatory arthropathies associated with ankylosing spondylitis, Reiter's syndrome, and inflammatory bowel diseases are also infrequent but well-established causes of SI-related pain. Intra-articular injection of the SI joint with local anesthetic and steroid can provide short-term pain relief and assist diagnostically in establishing the source of low back pain. Radiofrequency treatments for SI-related pain have been devised but are only modestly effective in a fraction of treated patients. A long-term solution to SI-related pain is one of the needs unmet by our current armamentarium.

Anatomy

The SI joints are paired structures formed by the sacrum medially and the ilium of the pelvis laterally. The SI joints are the principal load-bearing structures that connect the vertebral elements of the spine with the pelvis and lower extremities. The majority of the connection between the sacrum and the ilium is in the form of a dense fibrocartilaginous connection, rather than a true synovial joint. The bulk of the true joint space is limited to the anterior portion of the apposing surfaces of the SI connection. There is a small portion of the synovial joint space that extends to the

posterior- and inferior-most extent of the SI apposition, and it is from this point that access for intra-articular injection is gained. The superior extent of the SI joint lies anterior to the iliac crest, and the joint is difficult to access superior to the posterior-superior iliac spine (Fig. 8-1). The plane of the SI joint is variable from individual to individual; at the inferior extent of the joint where SI injection is carried out, the joint lies with 0 to 30 degrees of oblique angulation from the sagittal plane.

The sensory innervation to the SI joints is extensive, arising from branches of both the lumbar plexus anteriorly and the posterior sacral nerve roots posteriorly (the lateral branches of the posterior primary sacral rami from S1 to S4). Only the posterior aspect of the joint can be accessed with safety and ease percutaneously, and radiofrequency treatments have been devised to treat this portion of the SI joint.

Patient Selection

Patients with SI-related pain are difficult to distinguish from those with other causes of axial spinal pain, tending to report pain location over the SI joints to either side of midline near the lumbosacral junction (Fig. 8-2). Physical examination may reveal localized tenderness over the joint, and Patrick's test (or the Flexion, ABduction, External Rotation [FABER] test) may reproduce pain in the area of the SI joint positive (Table 8-1). Degenerative change of the joint on radiography is uncommon and nonspecific; most patients with SI-related pain have normal SI joint appearance on radiography. Resolution of pain following intra-articular injection of local anesthetic under fluoroscopic or computed tomography (CT) guidance is the best diagnostic tool available. Similar to facet joint pain, definitive diagnosis is hindered by the significant placebo effect of diagnostic injection. Treatment for SI joint pain remains inadequate and controversial. Currently, periodic intra-articular injection of steroid with local anesthetics is the most common therapy for SI joint pain but typically provides only transient relief.

Intra-articular Sacroiliac Joint Injection

Positioning

The patient lies prone, with the head turned to one side (Fig. 8-3). The c-arm is rotated 25 to 35 degrees caudally

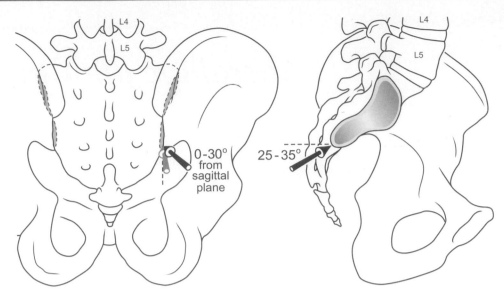

Figure 8-1.

Anatomy of the sacroiliac (SI) joints. The SI joints are largely stiff fibrocartilaginous connections, with the true synovial joint lying largely in the anterior aspect of the junction between the sacrum and the ilium. The true joint space extends to the inferior and posterior extent of the SI apposition, where it is accessible to injection. The plane of the posterior-inferior portion of the SI joint is variable, lying with 0 to 30 degrees of oblique angulation from the sagittal plane. The anterior portion of the joint arcs laterally. Accessing the joint is facilitated by a caudad-cephalad approach of 25 to 35 degrees to avoid the overlying posterior-superior iliac spine and iliac crest.

from the axial plane to place the posterior-superior iliac spine and the iliac crest cephalad along the line of the SI joint. The c-arm is then rotated obliquely 0 to 30 degrees until the posterior-inferior aspect of the SI joint is clearly visible (Fig. 8-4). Two features of the SI joint are important to recognize. First, the SI joint is curvilinear, often arcing somewhat laterally toward the anterior aspect. This can lead to confusing overlying shadows of the anterior and posterior portion of the joint (Figs. 8-4 and 8-5). The second important feature is the overlying iliac crest that can block entry to the SI joint (Fig. 8-6). To avoid placing a needle on the iliac crest rather than in the SI joint itself, use caudal angulation of the c-arm and limit injection to the inferior aspect of the joint.

Block Technique

The skin and subcutaneous tissues overlying the SI joint where the block is to be carried out are anesthetized with 1 to 2 mL of 1% lidocaine. A 22-gauge, 3.5-inch spinal needle is placed through the skin and advanced until it is seated in the tissues in a plane that is coaxial with the axis of the x-ray path (see Fig. 8-4). The needle is adjusted to remain coaxial or angled in a slightly cephalad direction toward the inferior aspect of the joint and advanced toward the joint space using repeat anterior-posterior images after every 2 to 4 mm of needle advancement. Once the surface of the joint space is contacted, the needle is advanced just slightly to

penetrate the posterior joint capsule. As the needle enters the joint space, the tip often curves slightly, following the contour of the surface of the ilium (see Fig. 8-4). In older patients and those with significant osteoarthritis, it may be difficult or impossible to penetrate into the joint space and only periarticular infiltration can be carried out. In most instances, there is no need for contrast injection to confirm needle location. The SI joint itself often holds only limited volume (typically <2 mL), and placing contrast in the joint limits the ability to place local anesthetic and steroid. A typical SI arthrogram is shown in Figure 8-7. A total dose of 80 mg of methylprednisolone acetate or the equivalent can be administered or divided between both SI joints if bilateral injection is necessary. Using concentrated steroid (40 or 80 mg per mL) allows 1:1 mixture with local anesthetic (0.5% bupivacaine) to provide immediate pain relief.

Complications of Intra-articular Sacroiliac Injection

Complications associated with intra-articular SI joint injection are uncommon. The most likely adverse effect is an exacerbation of pain in the days following resolution of the local anesthetic effect, likely owing to distention of the SI joint during the injection procedure. This exacerbation is usually mild and self-limited. Infection can also occur, leading to abscess within the presacral musculature, but the incidence is exceedingly low. Bleeding complications have not been associated with intra-articular SI injection.

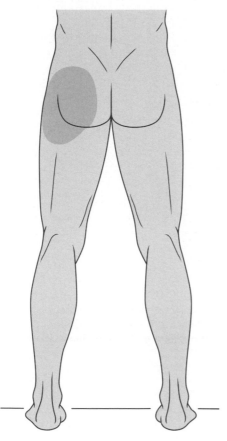

Figure 8-2.
Pattern of pain produced by sacroiliac (SI) joint dysfunction. The typical pain pattern produced by the SI joint is illustrated.

Radiofrequency Treatment of the Sacroiliac Joint

In those patients who receive only temporary relief from therapeutic intra-articular SI joint injections, there are limited treatment options available. Fusion of the joint is a major undertaking and has met with mixed results. In more recent years, several investigators have applied radiofrequency treatment to the SI joints in efforts to attain long-lasting pain relief. As discussed previously, the innervation to the SI joints arises from the lumbar plexus anteriorly, as well as the lateral branches of the posterior primary rami of the sacral nerve roots. It is not possible to denervate the entire joint using radiofrequency treatment, but denervation of the posterior portion of the joint can be affected by producing a striplike lesion along the posterior aspect of the joint, from the posterior-inferior portion of the joint cephalad to the posterior-superior iliac spine, the point where access to the joint is obstructed by the overlying iliac crest. Radiofrequency treatment of the lateral branch nerves of the posterior primary of the sacral nerve roots has also been described in preliminary reports. There is no single point of entry for the terminal sensory fibers to the SI joint, thus denervation is accomplished by creating a strip lesion along the posterior aspect of the joint capsule. This is done by using two radiofrequency cannulae positioned parallel to one another, no more than 5 to 6 mm apart along the posterior aspect of the joint. One of the two cannulae is attached to the electrode port of the radiofrequency generator, and the other cannula is attached to the ground (reference) port. The resulting lesion extends between the two cannulae (Fig. 8-8). By placing the cannulae sequentially one above the other along the posterior portion of the SI joint, a strip lesion is created. In limited case series, this treatment has shown significant efficacy (about one-third of patients will receive 50% or greater pain reduction lasting an average of 12 months).

Positioning

The patient lies prone, with the head turned to one side (see Fig. 8-3). The c-arm is rotated 25 to 35 degrees caudally from the axial plane to place the posterior-superior iliac spine and the iliac crest cephalad along the line of the SI joint. The c-arm is then rotated obliquely 0 to 30 degrees until the posterior-inferior aspect of the SI joint is clearly

---

Table 8–1

Provocative Tests for Sacroiliac Pain

Patrick's or FABER (Flexion, ABduction, External Rotation) test. The knee is flexed and the lateral malleolus of the ankle placed on the contralateral patella. The knee is then slowly lowered toward the examination table in external rotation. Pain caused by hip disease (e.g., osteoarthritis of the hip) is produced by this maneuver and is reported to radiate to the groin along the inguinal ligament. During the same maneuver, the examiner presses over the flexed knee while stabilizing the contralateral side of the pelvis over the anterior-superior iliac spine. This stresses the sacroiliac (SI) joint, and report of pain over the SI joint should raise suspicion of SI joint etiology.

Gaenslen's test. An alternate test for pain arising from the SI joint, Gaenslen's test, is performed by placing the patient supine along the edge of the examination table. One leg is placed over the edge of the examination table and lowered toward the floor in hyperextension while the pelvis is held stable. Pain related to the SI joint is reproduced by this maneuver.

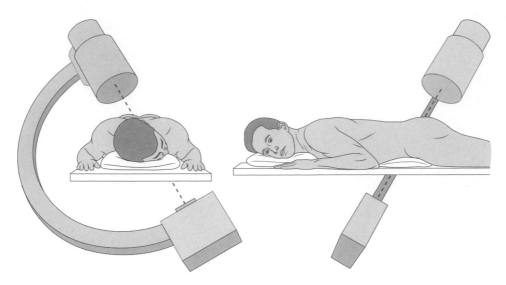

Figure 8-3.
Position for intra-articular sacroiliac joint injection. The patient is placed prone with the head turned to one side. The c-arm is angled 25 to 35 degrees caudally from the axial plane and 0 to 30 degrees obliquely until the posterior-inferior aspect of the joint is clearly visible.

visible (see Fig. 8-4). Two features of the SI joint are important to recognize. First, the SI joint is curvilinear, often arcing somewhat laterally toward the anterior aspect. This can lead to confusing overlying shadows of the anterior and posterior portion of the joint (see Figs. 8-4 and 8-5). The second important feature is the overlying iliac crest that can block access to the SI joint (see Fig. 8-6). Using caudal angulation of the c-arm and limiting injection to the inferior aspect of the joint are used to avoid placing a needle on the iliac crest rather than in the SI joint itself.

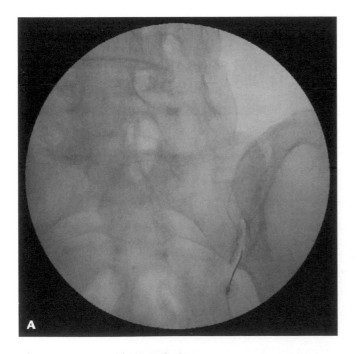
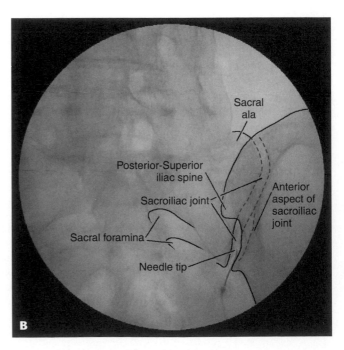

Figure 8-4.
Anterior-Posterior radiograph of the sacroiliac (SI) joint during intra-articular SI joint injection. **A:** A 22-gauge spinal needle is in position in the posterior-inferior aspect of the right SI joint. Note the medial deflection of the needle tip along the medial aspect of the ilium where the needle enters the joint space. **B:** Labeled image.

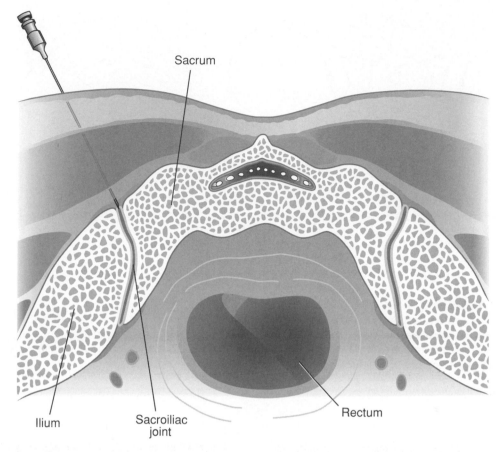

Sacrum

Ilium

Sacroiliac
joint

Rectum

Figure 8-5.
Axial diagram of intra-articular sacroiliac (SI) joint injection. The needle enters the posterior-inferior aspect of the SI joint. The anterior portion of the SI joint arcs laterally and can often be seen as a second line on radiographs that can be confused for the posterior aspect of the joint (see Fig. 8-4).

Block Technique

The skin and subcutaneous tissues overlying the SI joint where the block is to be carried out are anesthetized with 1 to 2 mL of 1% lidocaine. Three 10-cm SMK cannulae with 5-mm active tips are used for bipolar radiofrequency lesioning. The first cannula is placed at the inferior-most aspect of the joint, and then a second cannula is placed 5 to 6 mm above the first cannula (Fig. 8-9). Care should be taken to ensure the cannulae are at the same depth so the active tips lie nearly parallel to one another. The depth of placement should be to the surface of the SI joint capsule where an increase in resistance to needle advancement is first felt. Because there are no major sensory or motor nerves in the region, there is no need or use for sensory or motor testing during this procedure. After placing 0.5 mL of 2% lidocaine through each cannula, a bipolar lesion is created by treating at 90°C for 120 seconds. While the first lesion is being produced, a third cannula can be placed 5 to 6 mm cephalad to the second cannula, and local anesthetic instilled (see Fig. 8-9). After the first lesion is complete, the second

lesion can be started immediately. In this way, sequential lesions are created one above the other along the entire posterior and inferior aspect of the joint that is accessible. This usually results in a total of six to eight sequential lesions between the inferior pole of the joint and the point where further cephalad lesion creation is blocked by the posterior-superior iliac spine.

Complications of Radiofrequency Treatment of the Sacroiliac Joint

Patients should be warned of the typical postprocedural flare in pain symptoms that occurs after radiofrequency treatment of the SI joint. This results in an exacerbation of their typical pain lasting several days to a week. Major complications have not been reported with this radiofrequency procedure. Because there are no major nerves or blood vessels in the region, injury is unlikely. Similar to intra-articular injection, infection can also occur, leading to abscess within the presacral musculature; however, the incidence is exceedingly low.

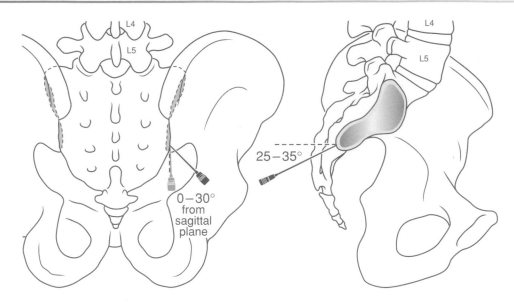

Figure 8-6.
Position and angle of needle entry for intra-articular sacroiliac (SI) joint injection. A 22-gauge spinal needle is advanced from 25 to 35 degrees caudad-cephalad to avoid the over-lying posterior-superior iliac spine. The axis of the SI joint varies from person to person with 0 to 30 degrees of oblique angulation.

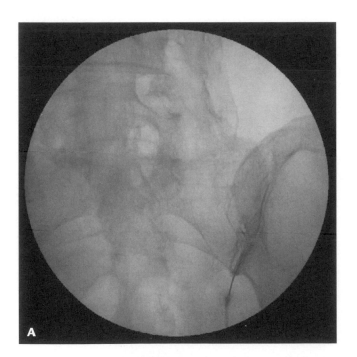

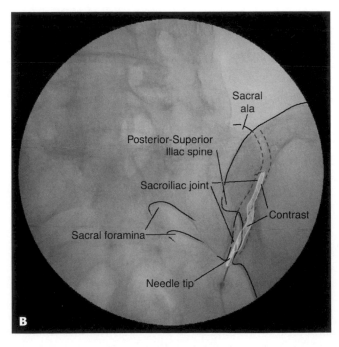

Figure 8-7.
Anterior-Posterior radiograph of the sacroiliac (SI) joint during intra-articular SI joint injection. **A:** A 22-gauge spinal needle is in position in the posterior-inferior aspect of the right SI joint, and 1.5 mL of radiographic contrast (iohexol 180 mg per mL) has been injected. Contrast extends to the superior portion of the joint. **B:** Labeled image.

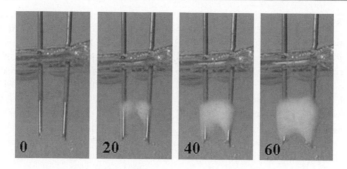

Figure 8-8.

Bipolar radiofrequency lesion. Two 10-cm SMK radiofrequency cannulae with 5-mm active tips are immersed in egg white, and a lesion is carried out at 90°C for 90 seconds. The lesion is maximal in size by 90 seconds of treatment and bridges between the two cannulae only if they remain less than 6 mm apart. If the cannulae are spaced more than 6 mm apart, two discrete unipolar lesions are created. (Preliminary data appear in Pino CA, Rathmell JP, Hofsess C et al. *Morphologic Analysis of Bipolar Radiofrequency Lesions: Implications for Denervation of the Sacroiliac Joint.* Presented at the annual fall meeting of the American Society of Regional Anesthesia and Pain Medicine, Phoenix, AZ, November 7–10, 2002.)

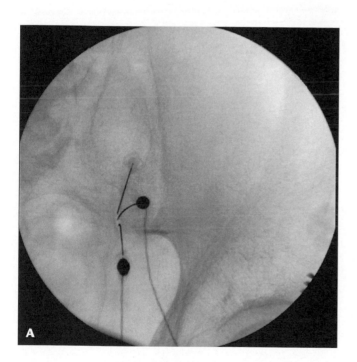
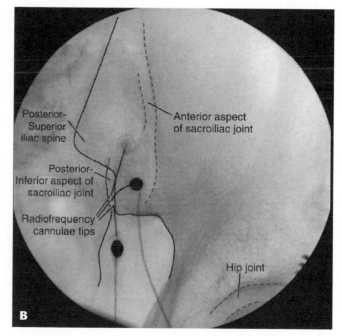

Figure 8-9.

Anterior-Posterior radiograph of the sacroiliac (SI) joint during bipolar radiofrequency treatment of the SI joint. **A:** Three separate 22-gauge, 10-cm SMK cannulae with 5-mm active tips are in position over the posterior-inferior aspect of the right SI joint. One of the cannulae is attached to the active electrode output from the radiofrequency generator, and the other is attached to the ground (reference electrode) port. Lesions are created at 90°C for 90 to 120 seconds. While the first lesion is being produced, a third cannula is placed within 6 mm cephalad to the second cannula. A second lesion is then created between the second and third cannulae, and additional cannulae are inserted just cephalad to the previous cannula along the entire posterior aspect of the SI joint. In this way, a series of connected lesions are created. The superior limit of the treatment is limited by access to the SI joint, which is blocked by the overlying posterior-superior iliac spine. **B:** Labeled image.

SUGGESTED READINGS

Calvillo O, Skaribas I, Turnipseed J. Anatomy and pathophysiology of the sacroiliac joint. *Curr Rev Pain*. 2000;4:356–361.

Carragee EJ, Hannibal M. Diagnostic evaluation of low back pain. *Orthop Clin North Am*. 2004;35:7–16.

Chou LH, Slipman CW, Bhagia SM et al. Inciting events initiating injection-proven sacroiliac joint syndrome. *Pain Med*. 2004;5:26–32.

Cohen SP, Abdi S. Lateral branch blocks as a treatment for sacroiliac joint pain: a pilot study. *Reg Anesth Pain Med*. 2003;28:113–119.

Dreyfuss P, Dreyer SJ, Cole A et al. Sacroiliac joint pain. *J Am Acad Orthop Surg*. 2004;12:255–265.

Ferrante FM, King LF, Roche EA et al. Radiofrequency sacroiliac joint denervation for sacroiliac syndrome. *Reg Anesth Pain Med*. 2001;26:137–142.

Luukkainen RK, Wennerstrand PV, Kautiainen HH et al. Efficacy of periarticular corticosteroid treatment of the sacroiliac joint in non-spondylarthropathic patients with chronic low back pain in the region of the sacroiliac joint. *Clin Exp Rheumatol*. 2002;20:52–54.

Schwarzer AC, Aprill CN, Bogduk N. The sacroiliac joint in chronic low back pain. *Spine*. 1995;20:31–37.

Young S, Aprill C, Laslett M. Correlation of clinical examination characteristics with three sources of chronic low back pain. *Spine J*. 2003;3:460–465.

CHAPTER 9

Lumbar Discography and Intradiscal Electrothermal Therapy

Overview

Discography is a diagnostic test in which radiographic contrast is injected into the nucleus pulposus of the intervertebral disc. Although originally developed for the study of disc herniation, discography is now used most commonly to identify symptomatic disc degeneration. There are two components of discography: (a) the anatomic appearance of contrast spread within the disc (using plain radiographs and/or computed tomography [CT]), and (b) the presence or absence of typical pain during contrast injection within the disc (pain provocation). The usefulness of discography remains controversial. Some clinicians routinely use discography to identify symptomatic discs prior to surgical fusion or intradiscal thermal annuloplasty, whereas others believe the test is of unproven benefit in identifying symptomatic discs. Discography remains the only test available that attempts to correlate pain response from the patient during provocation with abnormal discs discovered on imaging studies. Improved surgical outcomes following lumbar fusion have been reported when guided by the use of discography. Intradiscal electrothermal therapy (IDET) is a minimally invasive procedure that offers an alternative treatment to a subset of those patients with discogenic low back pain. Much like its use prior to fusion, discography is used to identify symptomatic intervertebral discs prior to IDET.

Anatomy

The intervertebral discs are comprised of glucosaminoglycans with a relatively fluid inner nucleus pulposus surrounded by a stiff, lamellar outer annulus fibrosis. With aging, the hydration of the intervertebral discs declines, leading to loss of disc height and fissure formation in the annulus fibrosis. These fissures begin centrally near the border between the nucleus pulposus and the annulus fibrosis, and can extend to the periphery of the disc space. This process of degradation is called internal disc disruption and is believed to be responsible for producing discogenic pain. These same radial fissures within the annulus represent paths through which nuclear material can pass and extrude as herniated nucleus pulposus. When this extruded material is adjacent to an exiting spinal nerve root, it can lead to intense inflammation, nerve root compression, and radicular pain with or without radiculopathy (nerve root dysfunction in the form of numbness, weakness, and/or loss of deep tendon reflexes).

The lowest three lumbar intervertebral discs (L3/L4, L4/L5, and L5/S1) are most commonly associated with discogenic pain. The disc spaces at these levels can be entered safely using an oblique approach by placing a needle that passes near the junction of the transverse process and the superior articular process of the vertebra bordering the inferior aspect of the disc space to be studied. The needle then passes medially and inferior to the exiting nerve root to penetrate the posterolateral aspect of the annulus en route to the center of the disc space (Fig. 9-1). The L3/L4 disc space lies close to the axial plane, whereas the plane of the L4/L5 and L5/S1 discs follow the lumbar lordosis and are angled progressively in a cephalad-caudal direction. A clear grasp of the plane in which each disc is typically found and accurate alignment of the c-arm are essential to carrying out discography safely and successfully.

Patient Selection

The patient with low back or neck pain originating from the vertebral disc often presents with deep, aching, axial midline pain. Pain can be referred to the buttocks and posterior thigh from lumber discs but does not extend to the distal extremities. Patients with discogenic pain are often young and otherwise healthy; discogenic pain is common in those with jobs that require repetitive motion of the affected spine segment (e.g., package handlers) or that expose the spine to excessive vibration (e.g., long-distance truck drivers, helicopter pilots, jackhammer operators). Onset of symptoms is usually gradual. Pain is experienced with prolonged sitting (sitting intolerance), standing, and bending forward.

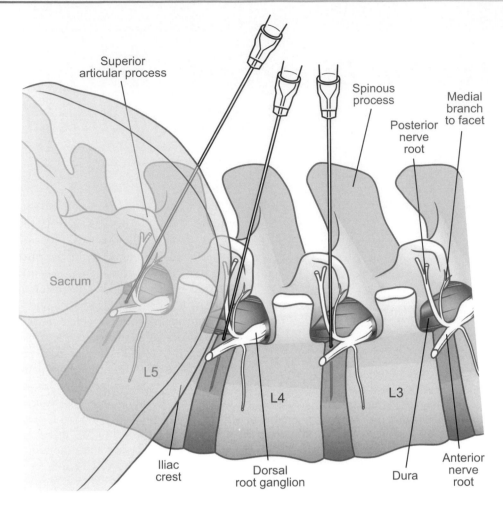

Figure 9-1.
Anatomy of the lumbar intervertebral discs (lateral view) during lumber discography. In general, the L3/L4 disc lies close to the axial plane, the L4/L5 disc is angled caudally 0 to 15 degrees, and the L5/S1 disc is angled caudally 25 to 35 degrees. Needles can be safely inserted into each disc through the posterolateral aspect of the annulus fibrosis, just caudal to the exiting nerve root.

The referred pain usually remains in the proximal part of the extremity. Results of physical examination are nonspecific, with limited range of motion at the affected segment, or pain with movement, particularly on flexion. Magnetic resonance imaging (MRI) and CT reveal only nonspecific findings, such as loss of disc height and/or hydration; these findings are often present without pain. The presence of a high-intensity zone on MRI at the posterior aspect of the disc indicates that a radial tear or fissure may be present in the annulus fibrosis, again a nonspecific finding commonly found in those without back pain. Treatment for discogenic pain starts with conservative therapy, including physical therapy and oral nonsteroidal anti-inflammatory drugs (NSAIDs). In those with prolonged or disabling pain that is suspected to be of discogenic origin, provocative discography can help identify the affected level and guide targeted therapy.

Diagnostic Lumbar Discography

Positioning

Lumbar discography is a painful procedure, even when performed by the most skilled practitioners. Intravenous sedation can facilitate the procedure; however, caution must be used to avoid over-sedation, which could impede ongoing communication with the patient. The patient must be able to report paresthesiae before neural injury occurs. Discography also relies on the patient to report the location and severity of symptoms during provocation, thus excessive sedation can make interpretation of the results difficult. The patient lies prone, with the head turned to one side (Fig. 9-2). A pillow is placed under the lower abdomen, above the iliac crest, in an effort to reduce the lumbar lordosis. Asking the patient to rotate the inferior aspect of the pelvis anteriorly toward the table will tip

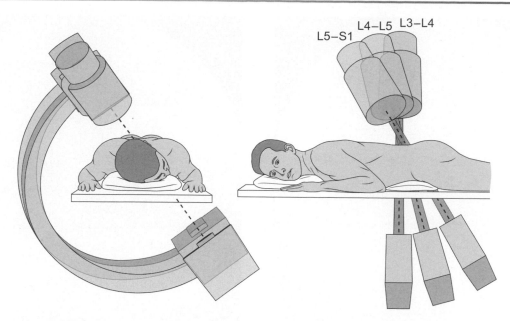

Figure 9-2.
Position for lumbar discography. The patient is placed prone with the head turned to one side. The c-arm is rotated 25 to 35 degrees obliquely and centered on the disc space to be studied. The c-arm is then angled in a cephalad direction that will vary from patient to patient, depending on the disc to be studied and each patient's degree of lumbar lordosis. In general, the L3/L4 disc lies close to the axial plane and requires no angulation to align the vertebral end plates, the L4/L5 disc requires 0 to 15 degrees of cephalad angulation, and the L5/S1 disc requires 25 to 35 degrees of cephalad angulation.

the iliac crest posteriorly and is often key to successfully performing discography at the L5/S1 level. The c-arm is rotated 25 to 35 degrees obliquely and centered on the disc space to be studied. The c-arm is then angled in a cephalad direction, the degree of which will vary from patient to patient, depending on the disc to be studied and each patient's degree of lumbar lordosis (see Fig. 9-2). In general, the L3/L4 disc lies close to the axial plane and requires no cephalad angulation to align the vertebral end plates (Fig. 9-3), the L4/L5 disc requires 0 to 15 degrees of cephalad angulation, and the L5/S1 disc requires 25 to 35 degrees of cephalad angulation (Fig. 9-4). Proper alignment of the c-arm is critical to the safety and success of discography.

Block Technique

The skin and subcutaneous tissues overlying the disc space where discography is to be carried out are anesthetized with 1 to 2 mL of 1% lidocaine, and additional local anesthetic is instilled liberally as the needle is advanced. A 22-gauge, 5-inch spinal needle is placed through the skin and advanced until it is seated in the tissues in a plane that is coaxial with the axis of the x-ray path (Figs. 9-3, 9-4, and 9-5). A 7- or 8-inch spinal needle is often required in obese patients and is often needed at

the L5/S1 level due to the long and oblique trajectory to the disc space. Without careful use of a coaxial technique throughout the entire course of needle advancement, discography will require redirecting the needle multiple times, if it can be done successfully at all. The direction of the needle should be rechecked after every 1 to 1.5 cm of needle advancement and adjusted to remain co-axial. The position of the exiting nerve root beneath the pedicle should be kept in mind at all times, and efforts to ensure the needle does not stray cephalad or lateral to the intended point over the middle of the disc will reduce the likelihood of striking the nerve root en route to the disc (Figs. 9-6 and 9-7). Once the needle is in contact with the surface of the disc, there will be a notable increase in resistance to needle placement. At this point, the c-arm should be rotated to a lateral position, and the needles should be advanced halfway from the anterior to the posterior margin of the disc (Fig. 9-8). Proper final placement is then checked in the anterior-posterior (AP) plane, where again the needle should be in the midportion of the disc space (Fig. 9-9). The nucleus pulposus occupies the central one-third of the disc space, and placement of the needle tip anywhere within the nucleus should suffice. The final needle path lies inferior to the exiting nerve root, and in many patients, it is difficult or impossible to position the needle exactly in the center of the disc (see Figs. 9-6 and 9-7).

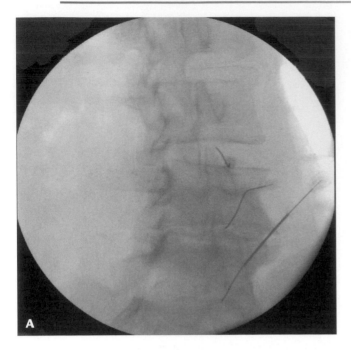

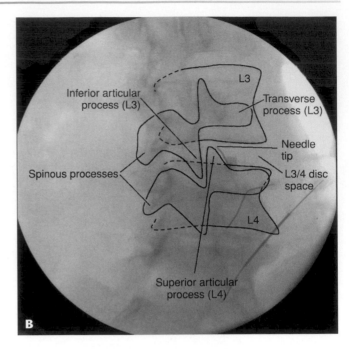

Figure 9-3.
Oblique radiograph during lumbar discography (L3/L4). **A:** The superior end plate of the L4 vertebral body is aligned with the inferior end plate of the L3 vertebral body. The junction of the L4 transverse process with the superior articular process lies just caudal to the L3/L4 disc space. A needle is directed slightly superior and posterior toward the L3/L4 disc space. The exiting L3 nerve root traverses inferior to the L3 pedicle and courses laterally, well superolateral to the path of the needle as it enters the disc space. **B:** Labeled figure.

Once the needles are in final position at all levels to be tested, provocative testing is conducted. A small volume of radiographic contrast containing antibiotic is placed at each level (<1.5 mL of iohexol 180 mg per mL containing 1 mg per mL of cefazolin). The contrast material is injected under live fluoroscopy to observe the pattern of contrast spread within the disc (Fig. 9-10). As the contrast is injected, the resistance to injection is noted and the patient is questioned about their symptoms. Some practitioners use an in-line pressure monitoring device to ensure excess pressure is not delivered during the provocative test. There is some evidence that pain reproduction using small volumes without excessive pressure during injection correlates most closely with symptomatic discogenic pain; injection under high pressure or with large volumes may well produce pain even in normal discs. A concordant discogram result occurs when the patient reports his or her typical pattern of severe pain during injection at the level of suspected pathology and the same patient reports no pain on injection of an adjacent disc that is normal in appearance. After injection of all levels, final AP and lateral radiographs should be obtained to document the levels tested and the patterns of contrast spread during injection. Some practitioners advocate for subsequent CT to assess the patterns of disc disruption using axial imaging (Figs. 9-11 and 9-12), but the usefulness of CT-discography in planning subsequent therapy is unclear.

Complications of Lumbar Discography

The majority of patients will experience a marked exacerbation of their typical back pain in the days following discography. They should be warned to expect this and given a short course of oral analgesics for treatment of the exacerbation. Less commonly, injury to the exiting nerve roots can occur. The position of the nerve roots is in close proximity to the needle's path (see Fig. 9-1). Care must be taken to advance the needle slowly as it passes over the transverse process en route to the posterolateral margin of the disc. If the patient reports a paresthesia to the lower extremity, the needle should be withdrawn and redirected. Paresthesia will occur in a small proportion of patients, even with good technique. Persistent paresthesiae are uncommon and typically ensue only after repeated paresthesiae occur during the procedure. Infection can also occur, leading to abscess within the presacral musculature, but the incidence is exceedingly low. Infection within the disc space (discitis) is the most feared complication of discography and occurs with an incidence of less than 1:1,000. Treatment of discitis may require long-term administration of intravenous antibiotics and/or the need for surgical removal of the infection. There have been no cases of discitis reported to date in patients who have received intradiscal antibiotics during discography. Bleeding complications have not been associated with intra-articular sacroiliac (SI) injection.

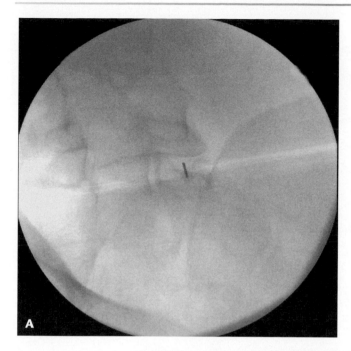

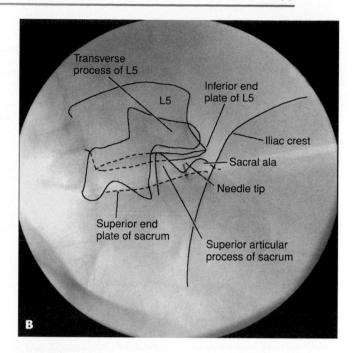

Figure 9-4.
Oblique radiograph during lumbar discography (L5/S1). **A:** The superior end plate of the sacrum is aligned with the inferior end plate of the L5 vertebral body. The junction of the sacral ala with the superior articular process of the sacrum lies just caudal to the L5/S1 disc space. The iliac crest overlies the anterior portion of the L5/S1 disc space, and its position often makes placing a needle for L5/S1 discography difficult. A needle is directed slightly superior toward the L5/S1 disc space. The exiting L5 nerve root traverses inferior to the L5 pedicle and courses laterally, just superolateral to the path of the needle as it enters the disc space. **B:** Labeled figure.

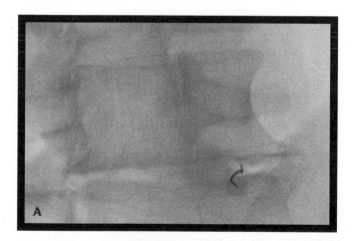

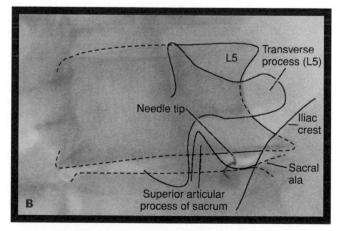

Figure 9-5.
Oblique radiograph during lumbar discography (L5/S1 in a patient with advanced disc degeneration and near complete loss of disc height). **A:** The superior end plate of the sacrum is aligned with the inferior end plate of the L5 vertebral body. Note the minimal remaining disc space: Discography can be difficult or impossible in those with minimal remaining disc height, and intradiscal treatments such as intradiscal electrothermal therapy should not be attempted unless disc height is well preserved. The junction of the sacral ala with the superior articular process of the sacrum lies just caudal to the L5/S1 disc space. The iliac crest overlies the anterior portion of the L5/S1 disc space, and its position often makes placing a needle for L5/S1 discography difficult. A needle is directed slightly superior toward the L5/S1 disc space. **B:** Labeled figure.

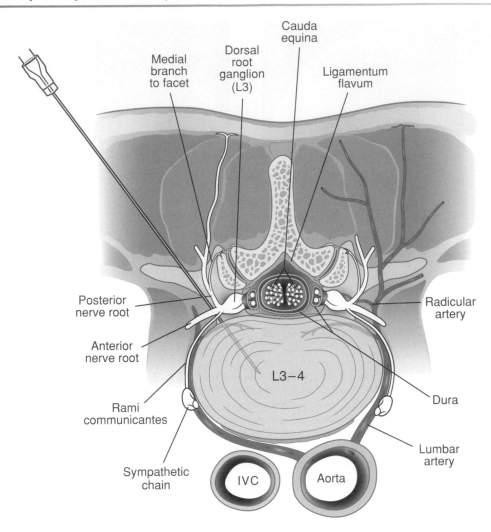

Medial branch to facet

Dorsal root ganglion (L3)

Cauda equina

Ligamentum flavum

Posterior nerve root

Radicular artery

Anterior nerve root

L3–4

Dura

Rami communicantes

Lumbar artery

Sympathetic chain

IVC   Aorta

Figure 9-6.
Axial diagram of L3/L4 discography. The needle enters the posterolateral aspect of the intervertebral disc, just inferomedial to the exiting L3 nerve root.

Intradiscal Electrothermal Therapy

In those patients who have early degenerative disc disease with preservation of near normal disc height (>75% of normal disc height remaining), but severe ongoing back pain that does not improve with conservative therapy, IDET (Smith & Nephew Orthopaedics, Memphis, TN) has appeared as a promising new treatment. Spinal fusion is usually reserved for those patients with more advanced disc degeneration. Patients who are suitable for IDET are those with concordant pain on discography at one or two spinal levels, and no pain during provocation of an adjacent control disc. IDET makes use of a navigable thermal resistance wire that is placed percutaneously and positioned along the posterior aspect of the of the annulus fibrosis (Fig. 9-13). Once in position, the disc is heated using a standardized protocol. Prospective studies have demonstrated significant pain reduction and improvement in physical function in 30% to 50% of patients who met these strict treatment criteria and who received IDET.

Positioning

Like discography, IDET is a painful procedure, even when performed by the most skilled practitioners. Intravenous sedation can facilitate the procedure, but a level of sedation that allows for ongoing communication with the patient is essential. The patient must be able to report paresthesiae or excess discomfort during the intradiscal treatment before neural injury occurs. Placement of the cannulae for IDET is identical to that for needle placement during discography. The patient lies prone, with the head turned to one side (see Fig. 9-2). A pillow is placed under the lower abdomen, above the iliac crest, in an effort to reduce the lumbar lordosis. The c-arm is rotated 25 to 35 degrees obliquely and centered on the disc space to be studied. The c-arm is then angled in a cephalad direction that will vary from patient to patient, depending on the disc to be studied and each patient's degree of lumbar lordosis (see Fig. 9-2). In general, the L3/L4 disc lies close to the axial plane and requires no cephalad angulation to align the vertebral end plates

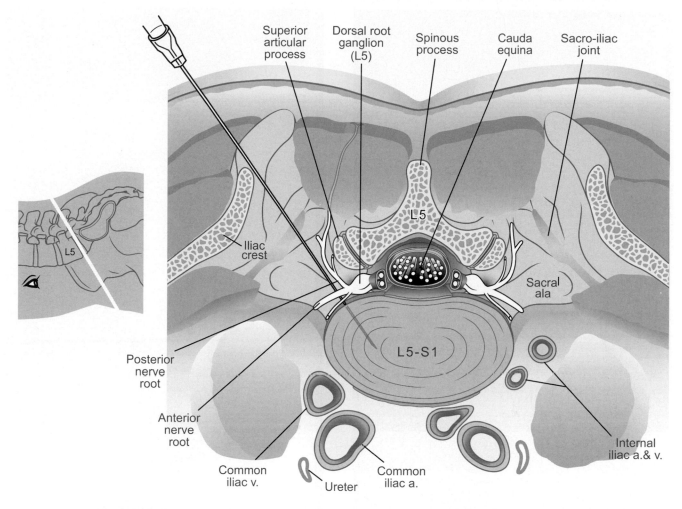

Figure 9-7.
Axial diagram of L5/S1 discography. The needle enters the posterolateral aspect of the intervertebral disc, just inferomedial to the exiting L5 nerve root. Note the position of the overlying iliac crest that often obscures direct needle placement. The inset indicates the approximate plane of the L5/S1 disc and needle.

(see Fig. 9-3), the L4/L5 disc requires 0 to 15 degrees of cephalad angulation, and the L5/S1 disc requires 25 to 35 degrees of cephalad angulation (see Fig. 9-4). Proper alignment of the c-arm is critical to the safety and success of IDET.

Block Technique

The technique for placing the cannulae through which the IDET catheter is introduced into the disc is similar to that for needle placement for discography. However, the final position of the introducer is best placed in the anterolateral aspect of the nucleus, rather than in the central portion of the nucleus. This allows for a more gradual angle as the IDET catheter exits the introducer and curves around the inner aspect of the annulus (see Fig. 9-13). The skin and subcutaneous tissues overlying the disc space where IDET is to be carried out are anesthetized with 1 to 2 mL of 1% lidocaine, and additional local anesthetic is instilled liberally as the cannulae are advanced. A 17-gauge

introducer supplied by the manufacturer is placed through the skin and advanced until it is seated in the tissues in a plane that is coaxial with the axis of the x-ray path (Fig. 9-14). The IDET introducer is stiff and easy to redirect as it is advanced. The direction of the cannula should be rechecked after ever 1 to 1.5 cm of needle advancement and adjusted to remain coaxial. The position of the exiting nerve root beneath the pedicle should be kept in mind at all times, and efforts to ensure the needle does not stray cephalad or lateral to the intended point over the middle of the disc will reduce the likelihood of striking the nerve root en route to the disc (see Figs. 9-6 and 9-7). Once the needle is in contact with the surface of the disc, there will be a notable increase in resistance to needle placement. At this point, the c-arm should be rotated to a lateral position, and the needles advanced halfway from the anterior to the posterior margin of the disc (Fig. 9-15). Proper final placement is then checked in the AP plane, where again the needle should be in the midportion of the disc space (Fig. 9-16).

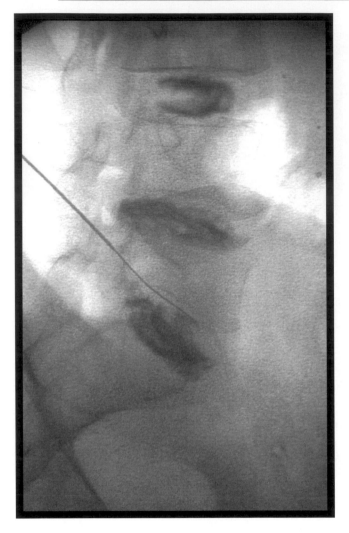

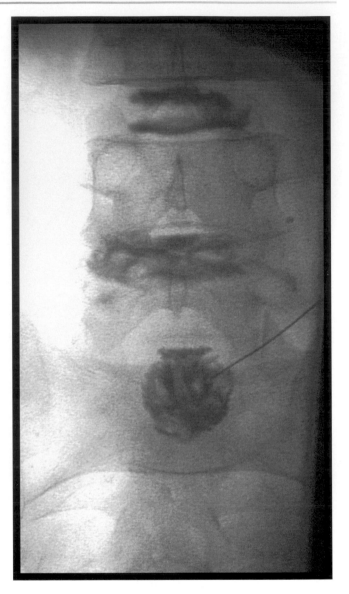

Figure 9-8.
Lateral radiograph of the lumbar spine following lumbar discography at the L3/L4, L4/L5, and L5/S1 levels. Disc height is normal at the L3/L4 level, markedly reduced at the L4/L5 level, and minimally reduced at the L5/S1 level. The L3/L4 discogram has the characteristic bilobed appearance of normal contrast spread within the nucleus pulposus, without any contrast extension into the annulus fibrosus. The L4/L5 discogram has diffuse linear spread of the dye to the limits of the annulus, with posterior extension of contrast into the epidural space. The L5/S1 discogram has a small extension of contrast into the annulus fibrosus posteriorly, but no extension into the epidural space. (Reprinted from Tarver JM, Rathmell JP, Alsofrom GF. Lumbar discography. *Reg Anesth Pain Med.* 2001;26:264, with permission.)

Figure 9-9.
Anterior-Posterior radiograph of the lumbar spine following lumbar discography at the L3/L4, L4/L5, and L4/S1 levels. Disc height is normal at the L3/L4 level, markedly reduced at the L4/L5 level, and minimally reduced at the L5/S1 level. The L3/L4 discogram has the characteristic bilobed appearance of normal contrast spread within the nucleus pulposus, without any contrast extension into the annulus fibrosus. The L4/L5 discogram has diffuse linear spread of the dye to the limits of the annulus fibrosus on both left and right sides. The L5/S1 discogram also appears normal. The circular appearance of the contrast is caused by the normal lumbar lordosis: The axis of the L5/S1 disc is tilted in a cephalad-to-caudad direction relative to the x-ray path. (Reprinted from Tarver JM, Rathmell JP, Alsofrom GF. Lumbar discography. *Reg Anesth Pain Med.* 2001;26:264, with permission.)

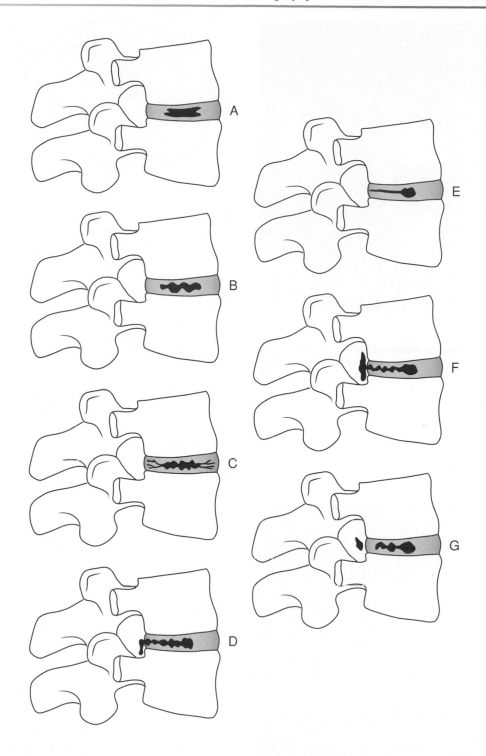

Figure 9-10.
Discogram morphology on the lateral projection. **A:** Normal. **B:** Degenerated disc.
C: Degenerated disc with an annular tear. **D:** Extruded disc (candle drip). **E:** Radial tear.
F: Radial tear with protruded disc. **G:** Extruded disc with a sequestered disc fragment.

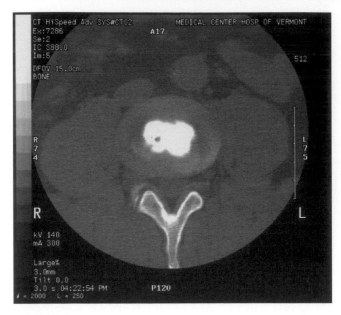

Figure 9-11.
Axial computed tomography image of a normal L3/L4 intervertebral disc following discography. Contrast is seen within the nucleus pulposus, without extension into the annulus fibrosus.

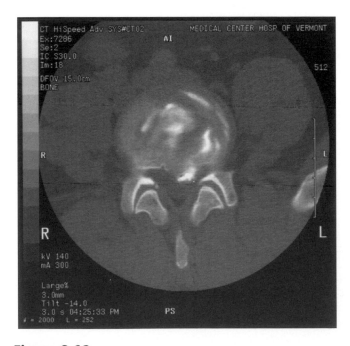

Figure 9-12.
Axial computed tomography image of an abnormal L4/L5 intervertebral disc following discography. Contrast is seen within the nucleus pulposus and extends into the annulus fibrosus in diffuse locations. Contrast is seen within a radial tear in the left posterolateral portion of the annulus and extends posteriorly into the epidural space.

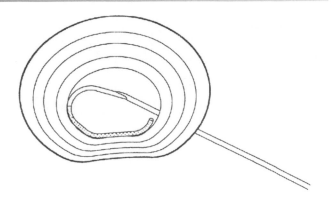

Figure 9-13.
Axial diagram of intradiscal electrothermal therapy introducer and catheter in proper position for treatment. The introducer is placed in the anterolateral portion of the nucleus pulposus. The catheter is then threaded through the introducer and steered along the inner circumference of the annulus fibrosis until the catheter is in place along the entire posterior annular wall. (Reprinted with permission of Smith & Nephew Orthopaedics, Memphis, TN.)

Once the IDET introducer is in a satisfactory position, the navigable thermal resistance catheter (SpineCATH, Smith & Nephew Orthopaedics, Memphis, TN) is introduced. The tip of the catheter slides along the medial circumference of the annulus and can be guided by gently rotating the proximal end of the catheter. The catheter is first advanced beyond the tip of the introducer and into the disc space using lateral radiography (see Fig. 9-15). When the tip of the catheter passes to the posterior aspect of the annulus and begins to traverse along the posterior annulus, the c-arm is then rotated to the AP view, and the catheter is advanced into final position across the entire posterior annulus (see Fig. 9-16). The catheter has two radiopaque guides that indicate the active treatment portion of the catheter, and these markers should be positioned to either side of the disc to indicate that the entire posterior annulus will be treated (see Fig. 9-16). This brief description is overly simplistic. In actuality, guiding the IDET catheter into final position can be quite challenging and requires delicate manipulation of the catheter to keep the tip from advancing into radial tears within the annulus. Overly aggressive handling of the catheter will cause it to kink, and once kinked, it will be difficult or impossible to steer.

Once the catheter is in final position, heat is introduced using a specific protocol designed to gradually raise the temperature within the disc to 80°C to 90°C and maintain that temperature for a minimum treatment period, typically 14 to 16 minutes. It is important that the patient is not overly sedated during the actual heat treatment so they can report discomfort due to excess heat, before neural injury occurs.

Complications of IDET

Patients should be warned of the typical postprocedural flare in pain symptoms that occurs after IDET. This results in an exacerbation of their typical axial back pain, often

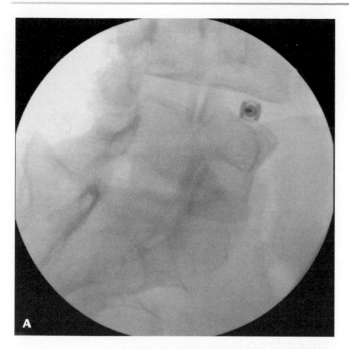
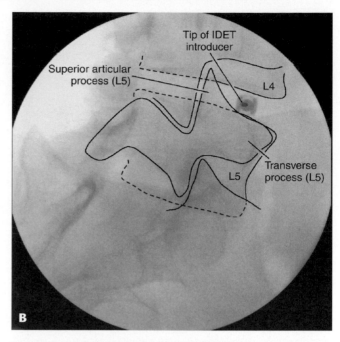

Figure 9-14.
Oblique radiograph of the lumbar spine demonstrating coaxial placement of the introducer cannula for intradiscal electrothermal therapy (IDET). **A:** The cannula is directed toward the anterolateral aspect of the L4/L5 intervertebral disc space. **B:** Labeled image.

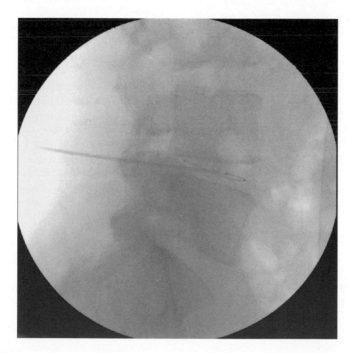

Figure 9-15.
Lateral radiograph of the lumbar spine during initial placement of the catheter for intradiscal electrothermal therapy (IDET). After the introducer is in position, the IDET catheter is threaded initially using radiographic guidance in the lateral view. In this plane, the IDET catheter can be followed as it hugs the contralateral inner annular wall and travels toward the posterior annular wall. When the tip of the cannula reaches the posterior annular wall, it should turn toward the ipsilateral side and hug the posterior annular wall. Great care should be taken to observe the position of the catheter along the posterior annular wall because, in the presence of a significant posterior annular tear, the catheter can easily exit the disc space and enter the epidural space.

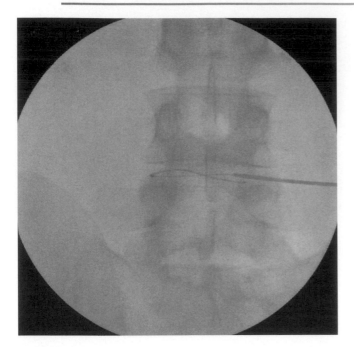

Figure 9-16.
Anterior-Posterior (AP) radiograph of the lumbar spine during final placement of the catheter for intradiscal electrothermal therapy (IDET). When the IDET catheter tip reaches the posterior annular wall in the lateral radiograph, the view is changed to the AP plane before the catheter is advanced further. The catheter is then guided across the posterior annular wall until the radiographic markers extend across the entire posterior annulus.

lasting several days to weeks. Less commonly, injury to the exiting nerve roots can occur. The position of the nerve roots is in close proximity to the needle's path (see Fig. 9-1). Care must be taken to advance the needle slowly as it passes over the transverse process en route to the posterolateral margin of the disc. If the patient reports a paresthesia to the lower extremity, the needle should be withdrawn and redirected. Paresthesia will occur in a small proportion of patients, even with good technique. Persistent paresthesiae are uncommon and typically ensue only after repeated paresthesiae occur during the procedure.

The key to successful outcome following IDET is strict adherence to a structured rehabilitation program that guides the patient through gradual increases in physical activity over a 6-week to 3-month time period. The rehabilitation following IDET is similar to the programs used following lumbar fusion. Thermal injury to the cauda equina has been reported following IDET with severe neuropathic pain in the lower extremities, as well as bowel and bladder dysfunction. Injury to the cauda equina is more likely to occur when there is an insufficient posterior annulus and the thermal catheter lies in close proximity to the thecal sac. The catheter can also exit the disc space to enter the epidural space; however, this should be evident before treatment on lateral radiographs. Ensuring the patient is awake enough to report excessive discomfort during the IDET treatment should reduce the chances of significant neural injury.

Finally, overly aggressive handling of the IDET catheter leads to kinking of the catheter near the point where it exits the tip of the introducer within the intervertebral disc. Repeated attempts to reposition the catheter once it is kinked can lead to shearing of the catheter tip.

SUGGESTED READINGS

Boden SD, Davis DO, Dina TS et al. Abnormal magnetic-resonance scans of the lumbar spine in asymptomatic subjects: a prospective investigation. *J Bone Joint Surg.* 1990;72:403–408.

Derby R, Howard MW, Grant JM et al. The ability of pressure-controlled discography to predict surgical and nonsurgical outcomes. *Spine.* 1999;24:364–372.

Guyer RD, Ohnmeiss DD. Contemporary concepts in spine care: lumbar discography. *Spine.* 1995;20:2,048–2,059.

Holt EP. The question of lumbar discography. *J Bone Joint Surg.* 1968; 50:720–726.

Lindblom K. Diagnostic puncture of intervertebral disks in sciatica. *Acta Orthop Scand.* 1948;17:213–239.

Pauza KJ, Howell S, Dreyfuss P et al. A randomized, placebo-controlled trial of intradiscal electrothermal therapy for the treatment of discogenic low back pain. *Spine J.* 2004;4:27–35.

Saal JA, Saal JS. Intradiscal electrothermal treatment for chronic discogenic low back pain. *Spine.* 2000;25:2,622–2,627.

Saal JA, Saal JS. Intradiscal electrothermal treatment for chronic discogenic low back pain: prospective outcome study with a minimum 2-year follow-up. *Spine.* 2002;27:966–973.

Stevens DS, Balatbat GR, Lee FMK. Coaxial imaging technique for superior hypogastric block. *Reg Anesth Pain Med.* 2000;24:643–647.

Tarver JM, Rathmell JP, Alsofrom GF. Lumbar discography. *Reg Anesth Pain Med.* 2001;26:263–266.

Tehranzadeh J. Discography 2000. *Radiol Clin North Am.* 1998;36: 463–495.

SYMPATHETIC AND PERIPHERAL NERVE BLOCKS

Stellate Ganglion Block

Overview

The sympathetic nervous system is involved in the pathophysiology that leads to a number of different chronic pain conditions, including complex regional pain syndrome (CRPS) and ischemic pain. These chronic pain states are often referred to as *sympathetically maintained pain* because they share the characteristic of pain relief following blockade of the regional sympathetic ganglia. Stellate ganglion block is an established method for the diagnosis and treatment of sympathetically maintained pain of the head, neck, and upper extremity.

Anatomy

Sympathetic fibers to and from the head, neck, and upper extremities pass through the stellate ganglion. In most individuals, the stellate ganglion is formed by fusion of the inferior cervical and first thoracic sympathetic ganglia. The ganglion is commonly found just lateral to the lateral border of the longus colli muscle, and anterior to the neck of the first rib and the transverse process of the seventh cervical vertebra (Figs. 10-1 and 10-2). In this position, the ganglion lies posterior to the superior border of the first part of the subclavian artery and the origin of the vertebral artery posterior to the dome of the lung. Although several approaches to stellate ganglion block have been described, the most common is the anterior paratracheal approach at C6 using surface landmarks. Performing the block at C6 reduces the likelihood of pneumothorax, which is more likely when the block is carried out close to the dome of the lung at C7. The anterior tubercle of the transverse process of C6 (Chassaignac's tubercle) is readily palpable in most individuals. To perform the block without radiographic guidance, the operator palpates the cricoid cartilage, and then slides a finger laterally into the groove between the trachea and the sternocleidomastoid muscle, retracting the muscle and adjacent carotid and jugular vessels laterally. Chassaignac's tubercle is typically palpable in this groove at the C6 level. Once the tubercle has been identified, a needle is advanced through the skin and seated on the tubercle, where local anesthetic is injected. The local anesthetic spreads along the prevertebral fascia in a caudal direction to anesthetize the stellate ganglion, which lies just inferior to the point of injection in the same plane. In practice, there is marked variation in the size and shape of Chassaignac's tubercle that reduces the rate of successful block. The adjacent vertebral artery and C6 nerve root must be avoided to safely conduct this block (Figs. 10-1 to 10-3). A simple modification of technique in which the needle is directed medially toward the base of the transverse process using radiographic guidance is a safe and simple means of improving the reliability of stellate ganglion block and is described in the following sections.

Patient Selection

Stellate ganglion block has long been the standard approach to diagnosis and treatment of sympathetically maintained pain syndromes involving the upper extremity, such as CRPS. Other neuropathic pain syndromes, including ischemic neuropathies, herpes zoster (shingles), early postherpetic neuralgia, and postradiation neuritis may also respond to stellate ganglion block. Blockade of the stellate ganglion has also proven successful in reducing pain and improving blood flow in vascular insufficiency conditions such as intractable angina pectoris, Raynaud's disease, frostbite, vasospasm, and occlusive and embolic vascular disease. Finally, the sympathetic fibers control sweating; thus, stellate ganglion block can be quite effective in controlling hyperhidrosis (recurrent and uncontrollable sweating of the hands).

Causalgia (CRPS, type 2) was first described during the American Civil War. Soon thereafter, it was recognized that blockade of the sympathetic chain with local anesthetic could produce significant pain relief in patients with causalgia. Patients with CRPS have a history of trauma to the affected area: Those with a major nerve trunk injury, such as a gunshot wound to the brachial plexus, are classified as CRPS, type 2 (causalgia), and those with no major nerve trunk injury are classified as CRPS, type 1 (reflex sympathetic dystrophy). Both types of CRPS share the same signs and symptoms. Patients with CRPS report pain that has characteristics of

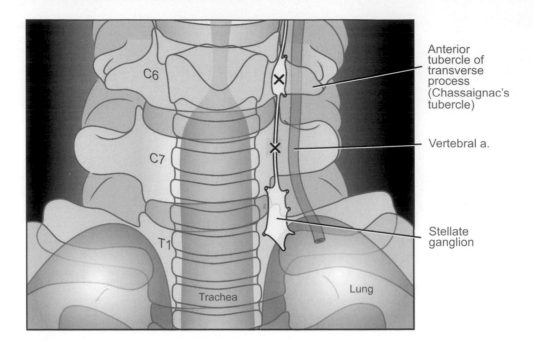

Figure 10-1.
Anatomy of the stellate ganglion. The stellate ganglion conveys sympathetic fibers to and from the upper extremities and the head and neck. The ganglion is comprised of the fused superior thoracic ganglion and the inferior cervical ganglion and is named for its fusiform shape (in many individuals, the two ganglia remain separate). The stellate ganglia lie over the head of the first rib at the junction of the transverse process and uncinate process of T1. The ganglion is just posteromedial to the cupola of the lung and medial to the vertebral artery. Stellate ganglion block is typically carried out at the C6 or C7 level to avoid pneumothorax, and a volume of solution that will spread along the prevertebral fascia inferiorly to the stellate ganglion is employed (usually 10 mL). When radiographic guidance is not used, the operator palpates the anterior tubercle of the transverse process of C6 (Chassaignac's tubercle), and a needle is seated in this location. With radiographic guidance, it is simpler and safer to place a needle over the vertebral body just inferior to the uncinate process of C6 or C7. Particular care should be taken when performing the block at the C7 level to ensure the needle does not stray lateral to the uncinate process because the vertebral artery courses anterior to the transverse process at this level and is often not protected within a bony foramen transversarium. The Xs mark the target for needle placement when performing stellate ganglion block at either the C6 or C7 level.

neuropathic pain, including spontaneous burning pain and allodynia (pain produced by stimulation that usually does not cause pain, such as light touch). Patients with CRPS also report symptoms or have signs on physical examination of sympathetic dysfunction. These include temperature and color asymmetries between the affected and unaffected limbs, edema, and asymmetries in sweating of the limbs. Dystrophic changes may appear late in the course of CRPS, including thinning of the skin, hair loss, and pitting of the nail beds.

Patients with signs and symptoms of CRPS may gain significant pain relief from stellate ganglion block. Unfortunately, the duration and magnitude of the pain relief are unpredictable. This led to the use of repeated sympathetic blocks, sometimes as often as daily or weekly blocks over an extended period of time in an attempt to improve the duration of pain relief. Experts widely agree that repeated sympathetic blocks alone rarely eliminate the pain and disability associated with CRPS. Incorporating sympathetic blockade

into a coordinated, multidisciplinary rehabilitation plan is essential for effective treatment of patients with CRPS. This treatment plan typically includes physical therapy, oral neuropathic pain medications, and supportive psychotherapy. Neuroablation has been used to destroy the sympathetic chain in those patients who attain excellent pain relief of temporary duration with local anesthetic blocks. There are few data available to evaluate the success of sympathetic ablation, and expert opinion is varied regarding the usefulness of this approach in the long-term treatment of CRPS.

Positioning

The patient lies supine, facing directly forward with a pillow under the upper back and lower neck to hold the neck in a slight extension (Fig. 10-4). The c-arm is centered over the lower cervical spine without angulation. The position of

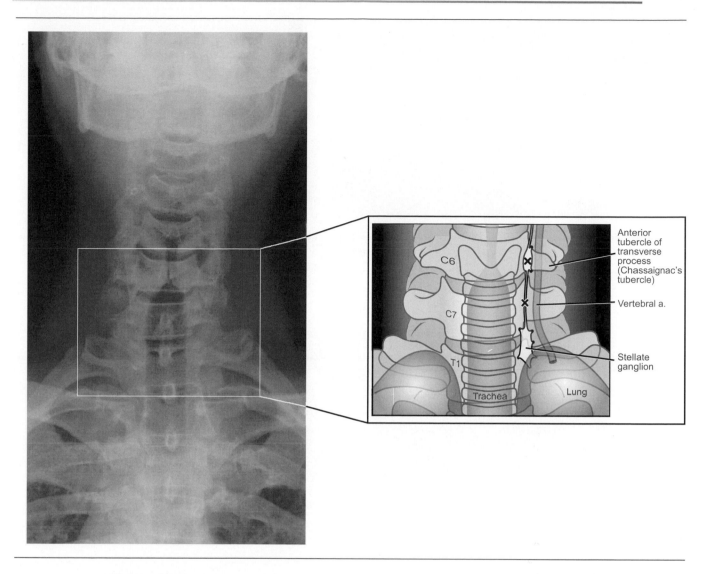

Figure 10-2.
Correlation between position of the stellate ganglion, the vertebral artery, and the inferior cervical vertebrae. The relative positions of the C6, C7, and T1 vertebral bodies; Chassaignac's tubercle (anterior tubercle of C6 transverse process); and the vertebral artery are illustrated. The vertebral artery traverses within the bony foramen transversarum at the C6 level, but the presence of a bony foramen at C7 is variable, and here the artery often courses unprotected anterior to the C7 transverse process. (Adapted from Janik JE, Hoeft MA, Rathmell JP. *Anatomic variation of Chassaignac's tubercle measured by computed tomography: implications for stellate ganglion block.* Presented at the annual fall meeting of the American Society of Regional Anesthesia and Pain Medicine, Phoenix, AZ, November 7–10, 2002.)

the vertebral bodies and transverse processes of C6 and C7 are identified (see Fig. 10-2).

Block Technique

The skin and subcutaneous tissues overlying the base of the transverse process of C6 or C7 on the affected side are anesthetized with 1 to 2 mL of 1% lidocaine. The transverse processes are often difficult to distinguish from the underlying facet columns, but the transverse process joins the vertebral body just inferior to the uncinate process of the vertebral body, a structure that is easy discernible on the

posterior-anterior radiograph (Fig. 10-5). The block can be carried out at either the C6 or the C7 level when using radiographic guidance. However, it is important to realize that the vertebral artery overlies the base of the transverse process at C7, and many individuals lack a bony foramen transversarum at this level (see Figs. 10-1 and 10-2). Thus, at C7, care must be taken to keep the needle tip in line or medial to a line connecting the uncinate process of C7 and T1. Straying more lateral will risk penetration of the vertebral artery. The overlying carotid artery must be retracted laterally to perform the classic technique for stellate ganglion block over the C6 transverse process, but this is unnecessary when the needle is directed toward the base of the transverse process

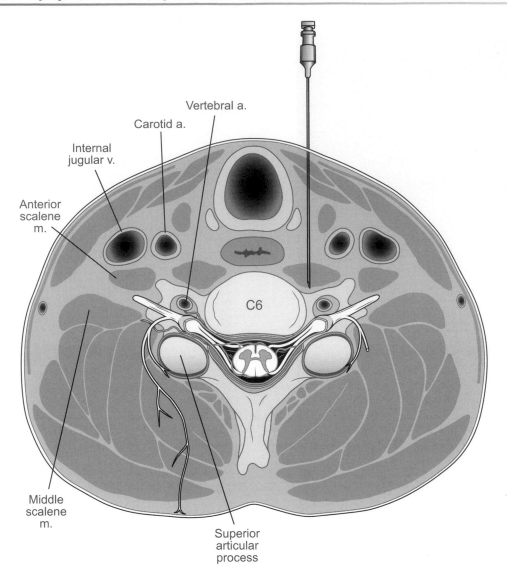

Vertebral a.

Carotid a.

Internal
jugular v.

Anterior
scalene
m.

C6

Middle
scalene
m.

Superior
articular
process

Figure 10-3.
Axial diagram of stellate ganglion block. The needle is positioned in the vertebral gutter, a
shallow depression where the transverse process joins with the vertebral body. Note the
position of the vertebral artery within the foramen transversarum, the exiting nerve root,
and the carotid artery.

(see Fig. 10-3). A 25-gauge, 3-inch needle is placed through the skin and advanced until it is seated in the tissues in a plane that is coaxial with the axis of the x-ray path. The needle may not remain seated easily without advancing the needle further than is safe before checking the needle's direction with fluoroscopy. The needle can be held in a coaxial plane using a small clamp or hemostat and directed toward the target in this manner. The needle is adjusted to remain coaxial as it is directed toward the base of the transverse process, just inferior to the uncinate process using repeat posterior-anterior (PA) images after every 2 to 4 mm of needle advancement. Once the surface of the vertebral body is contacted, the needle is in final position. Intravascular placement is ruled out and proper position is ensured by injecting 1 to 1.5 mL of radiographic contrast (iohexol 180 mg per mL or the equivalent). The contrast should spread

along the anterolateral margin of the vertebral bodies in both PA and lateral radiographs (Figs. 10-5 to 10-7). Thereafter, 10 mL of local anesthetic (0.25% bupivacaine) are injected incrementally. Repeat radiographs following local anesthetic injection should show dilution of the contrast and spread of the solution inferior to the T1 level where the stellate ganglion lies. Sympathetic block should ensue within 20 minutes following injection and is ensured by seeing a 1°C or greater rise in temperature of the ipsilateral hand. Signs of successful stellate ganglion block are listed in Table 10-1.

Complications

There are many structures within the immediate vicinity of the needle's tip once it is properly positioned for stellate ganglion block (see Figs. 10-1 and 10-3). Commonly, diffusion of

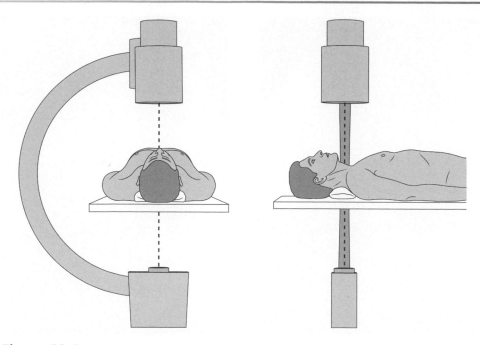

Figure 10-4.
Position for stellate ganglion block. The patient lies supine with a pillow beneath the upper back and lower neck to place the neck in slight extension. The c-arm is positioned over the cervicothoracic junction without angulation.

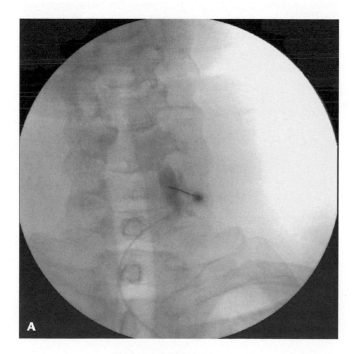

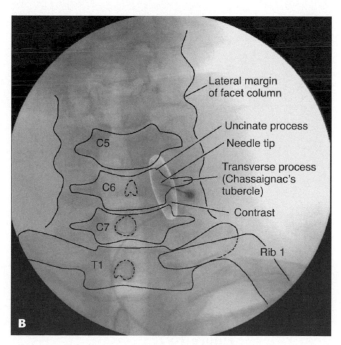

Figure 10-5.
Posterior-Anterior radiograph of the cervical spine during stellate ganglion block at C6. **A:** The needle is in position at the junction of the C6 transverse process and the vertebral body, just inferior to the uncinate process of C6. Radiographic contrast (1.5 mL of iohexol 180 mg per mL) has been injected and spreads along the anterolateral surface of C6 to reach the adjacent vertebra. Typically, 5 to 10 mL of volume are necessary to see spread to the level of the stellate ganglion at T1. **B:** Labeled image.

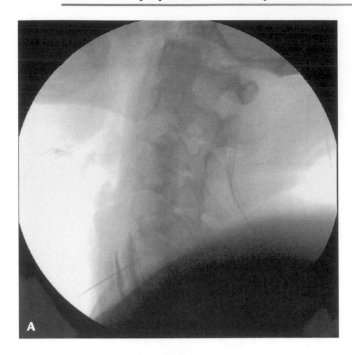
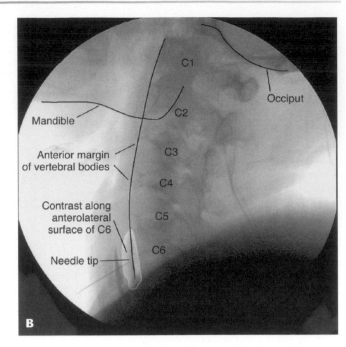

Figure 10-6.

Lateral radiograph of the cervical spine during stellate ganglion block at C6. **A:** The needle is seated against the anterior surface of C6. Radiographic contrast (1.5 mL of iohexol 180 mg per mL) has been injected and spreads along the anterolateral surface of C6 to reach the adjacent vertebra. A small amount of contrast is seen in a more superficial plane and was placed before the needle was firmly seated against the vertebral body. **B:** Labeled image.

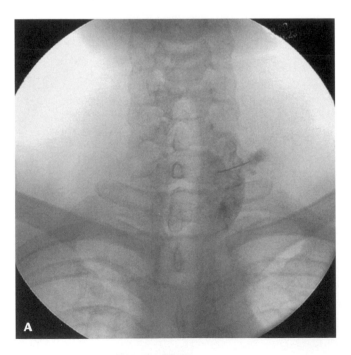
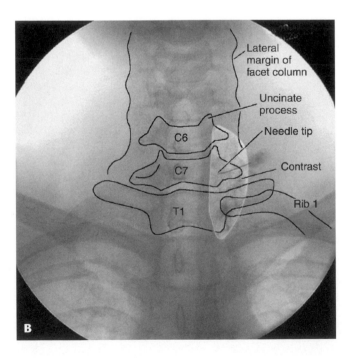

Figure 10-7.

Posterior-Anterior radiograph of the cervical spine during stellate ganglion block at C7. **A:** The needle is in position at the junction of the C7 transverse process and the vertebral body, just inferior to the uncinate process of C7. Particular care must be taken when performing stellate ganglion block at the C7 level. The needle tip must remain aligned below the uncinate process or more medial to avoid the vertebral artery, which courses unprotected over the anterior surface of the C7 transverse process in many individuals. Radiographic contrast (1.5 mL of iohexol 180 mg per mL) has been injected, followed by 10 mL of 0.25% bupivacaine, and spreads along the anterolateral surface of C6 to T2. **B:** Labeled image.

Table 10–1
Signs of Successful Stellate Ganglion Block

• Horner's syndrome
  • Miosis (pupillary constriction)
  • Ptosis (drooping of the upper eyelid)
  • Enophthalmos (recession of the globe within the orbit)
• Anhidrosis (lack of sweating)
• Nasal congestion
• Venodilation in the hand and forearm
• Increase in temperature of the blocked limb by at least 1°C

local anesthetic blocks the adjacent recurrent laryngeal nerve. This often leads to hoarseness, a feeling of having a lump in the throat, and a subjective feeling of shortness of breath and difficulty swallowing. Bilateral stellate ganglion block should not be performed because bilateral recurrent laryngeal nerve blocks may well lead to loss of laryngeal reflexes and respiratory compromise. The phrenic nerve is also commonly blocked by direct spread of local anesthetic and will lead to unilateral diaphragmatic paresis. Diffusion of local anesthetic, as well as direct placement of local anesthetic adjacent to the posterior tubercle, will result in somatic block of the upper extremity. This may take the form of a small area of sensory loss due to diffusion of local anesthetic or a complete brachial plexus block when the local anesthetic is placed within the nerve sheath. Patients with significant somatic block to the upper extremity should be sent home with a sling in place and counseled to guard their limb, just as one would instruct a patient who had received a brachial plexus block.

Major complications associated with stellate ganglion block include neuraxial block (spinal or epidural) and seizures. Extreme medial angulation of the needle from a relatively lateral skin entry point may lead to needle placement into the spinal canal through the anterolaterally oriented intervertebral foramen. In this manner, local anesthetic can be deposited in the epidural space or, if the needle is advanced far enough, it may penetrate the dural cuff surrounding the exiting nerve root and lie within the intrathecal space. More likely is placement of the needle tip on the posterior tubercle of the transverse process and spread of local anesthetic proximally along the nerve root to enter the epidural space. In this case, partial or profound neuraxial block, including high spinal or epidural block with loss of consciousness and apnea may ensue. Airway protection, ventilation and intravenous sedation should be promptly administered and continued until the patient regains airway reflexes and consciousness. Because the maximal effects of epidural local anesthetic may require 15 to 20 minutes to develop when using longer-acting local anesthetics, it is imperative that patients are monitored for at least 30 minutes after stellate ganglion block.

Intravascular injection during stellate ganglion block will likely result in immediate onset of generalized seizures. The carotid artery lies just anteromedial to Chassaignac's tubercle, whereas the vertebral artery lies within the bony transverse foramen just posteromedial to the tubercle. If injection occurs into either structure, the local anesthetic injected enters the arterial supply traveling directly to the brain, and generalized seizures typically begin rapidly and after only small amounts of local anesthetic (as little as 0.2 mL of 0.25% bupivacaine have led to seizure). However, because the local anesthetic rapidly redistributes, the seizures are typically brief and do not require treatment. In the event of seizure, halt the injection, remove the needle, and begin supportive care (see Chapter 4 for more detail regarding local anesthetic toxicity).

SUGGESTED READINGS

Brown DL. *Atlas of Regional Anesthesia.* 2nd ed. Philadelphia: WB Saunders; 1999:187–194.

Lamer TJ. Sympathetic nerve blocks. In: Brown DL, ed. *Regional Anesthesia and Analgesia.* Philadelphia: WB Saunders; 1996:357–384.

Rathmell JP. Sympathetic blocks. In: Rathmell JP, Neal JM, Viscomi CV, eds. *Requisites in Anesthesiology: Regional Anesthesia.* Philadelphia: Elsevier Health Sciences: 2004:128–141.

Rauck R. Sympathetic nerve blocks: head, neck, and trunk. In: Raj PP, ed. *Practical Management of Pain.* 3rd ed. St. Louis, MO: Mosby; 2000:651–682.

Celiac Plexus Block and Neurolysis

Overview

Neurolytic celiac plexus block (NCPB) is among the most widely applicable of all neurolytic blocks. NCPB has a long-lasting benefit for 70% to 90% of patients with pancreatic and other intra-abdominal malignancies. Several techniques have been described for localizing the celiac plexus. The classic technique employs a percutaneous posterior approach, using surface and bony landmarks to position needles in the vicinity of the plexus. Numerous reports have described new approaches for celiac plexus block, using guidance from plain radiographs, fluoroscopy, computed tomography (CT), or ultrasound. No single methodology has proven clearly superior in either its safety or its success rate. In more recent years, it has been generally agreed that radiographic guidance is necessary to perform celiac plexus block. Many practitioners have turned to routine use of CT, taking advantage of the ability to visualize adjacent structures when performing this technique.

Anatomy

The celiac plexus is comprised of a diffuse network of nerve fibers and individual ganglia that lie over the anterolateral surface of the aorta at the T12/L1 vertebral level. Sympathetic innervation to the abdominal viscera arises from the anterolateral horn of the spinal cord between the T5 and T12 levels. Nociceptive information from the abdominal viscera is carried by afferents that accompany the sympathetic nerves. Presynaptic sympathetic fibers travel from the thoracic sympathetic chain toward the ganglion, traversing over the anterolateral aspect of the inferior thoracic vertebrae as the greater (T5 to T9), lesser (T10 to T11), and least (T12) splanchnic nerves (Fig. 11-1). Presynaptic fibers traveling via the splanchnic nerves synapse within the celiac ganglia over the anterolateral surface of the aorta surrounding the origin of the celiac and superior mesenteric arteries at approximately the L1 vertebral level. Postsynaptic fibers from the celiac ganglia innervate all the abdominal viscera, with the exception of the descending colon, sigmoid colon, rectum, and pelvic viscera.

Celiac plexus block using a transcrural approach places the local anesthetic or neurolytic solution directly on the celiac ganglion anterolateral to the aorta (see Fig. 11-1). The needles pass directly through the crura of the diaphragm en route to the celiac plexus. Spread of the solution toward the posterior surface of the aorta may thus be limited, perhaps reducing the chance of nerve root or spinal segmental artery involvement. In contrast, splanchnic nerve block (see Fig. 11-1) avoids the risk of penetrating the aorta and uses smaller volumes of solution, and the success is unlikely to be affected by anatomic distortion caused by extensive tumor or adenopathy within the pancreas. Because the needles remain posterior to the diaphragmatic crura in close apposition to the T12 vertebral body, this has been termed the retrocrural technique. Splanchnic nerve block is a minor modification of the classic retrocrural celiac plexus block; the only difference being that for splanchnic block, the needles are placed over the midportion of the T12 vertebral body rather than over the cephalad portion of L1. Retrocrural celiac plexus block at the superior aspect of the L1 vertebral body and splanchnic nerve block at the mid T12 vertebral body have both been described, and they are essentially the same technique, relying on cephalad spread of solution to block the splanchnic nerves in a retrocrural location. In most cases, celiac plexus (transcrural or retrocrural) and splanchnic nerve block can be used interchangeably to affect the same results. Although there are those who strongly advocate one approach over the other, there is no evidence that either results in superior clinical outcomes.

Patient Selection

Celiac plexus and splanchnic nerve block are used to control pain arising from intra-abdominal structures. These structures include the pancreas, liver, gall bladder, omentum, mesentery, and alimentary tract from the stomach to the transverse colon. The most common application of NCPB is to treat pain associated with intra-abdominal malignancy, particularly pain associated with pancreatic

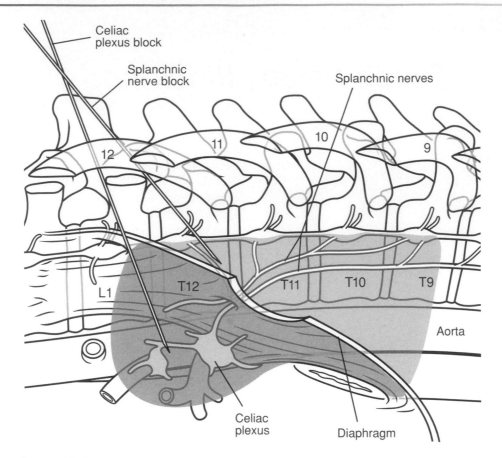

Figure 11-1.

Anatomy of the celiac plexus and splanchnic nerves. The celiac plexus is comprised of a diffuse network of nerve fibers and individual ganglia that lie over the anterolateral surface of the aorta at the T12/L1 vertebral level. Presynaptic sympathetic fibers travel from the thoracic sympathetic chain toward the ganglion, traversing over the anterolateral aspect of the inferior thoracic vertebrae as the greater (T5 to T9), lesser (T10 to T11), and least (T12) splanchnic nerves. Celiac plexus block using a transcrural approach places the local anesthetic or neurolytic solution directly on the celiac ganglion anterolateral to the aorta. The needles pass directly through the crura of the diaphragm en route to the celiac plexus. In contrast, for splanchnic nerve blocks the needles remain posterior to the diaphragmatic crura in close apposition to the T12 vertebral body. Shading indicates the pattern of solution spread for each technique.

cancer. Neurolysis of the splanchnic nerves or celiac plexus can produce dramatic pain relief, reduce or eliminate the need for supplemental analgesics, and improve quality of life in patients with pancreatic cancer and other intra-abdominal malignancies. The long-term benefit of NCPB in patients with chronic nonmalignant pain, particularly those with chronic pancreatitis, is debatable.

Positioning

The patient lies prone with the head turned to one side (Fig. 11-2). The c-arm is centered over the thoracolumbar junction. The final needle position for celiac plexus block is over the anterolateral surface of the aorta, just anterior to the T12/L1 junction. The c-arm is rotated obliquely 20 to

30 degrees, until the tip of the transverse process of L1 overlies the anterolateral margin of the L1 vertebral body (Fig. 11-3). The final needle position for splanchnic nerve block is anterolateral to the T12 vertebral body; thus, cephalad angulation of the c-arm is also needed to bring the inferior margin of the twelfth rib cephalad to the T12 vertebral body (see Fig. 11-2).

Block Technique

Celiac Plexus Block (Transcrural Technique)

Once the c-arm is aligned, the skin and subcutaneous tissues overlying the superior margin of the L1 vertebral body are anesthetized with 1 to 2 mL of 1% lidocaine. The aorta lies to the left of midline over the vertebral bodies. By routinely

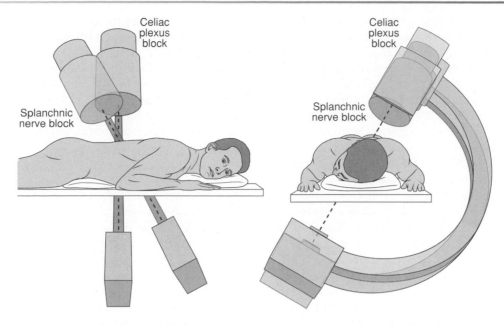

Figure 11-2.
Position for celiac plexus block and splanchnic nerve block. The patient is placed prone with the head turned to one side. The c-arm is rotated obliquely 20 to 30 degrees until the tip of the transverse process of L1 overlies the anterolateral margin of the L1 vertebral body (Fig. 11-3). For splanchnic nerve block, the c-arm is then angled 20 to 30 degrees cephalad to bring the inferior margin of the twelfth rib cephalad to the T12 vertebral body.

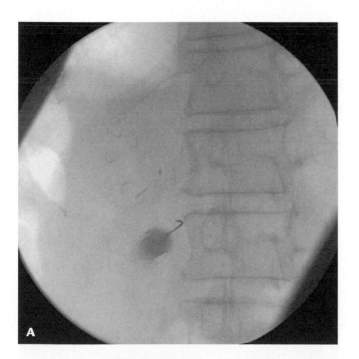
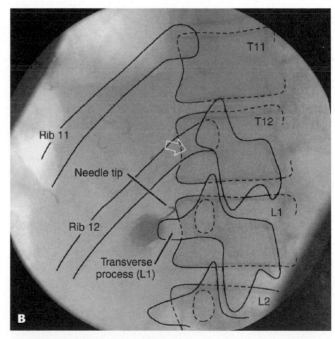

Figure 11-3.
Oblique radiograph of the spine during celiac plexus block. **A:** A needle passes from left oblique angle to lie over the anterolateral surface of the superior aspect of the L1 vertebral body. It passes superior to the transverse process of L1 and inferomedial to the twelfth rib. **B:** Labeled image. The white arrow indicates the final needle position for splanchnic nerve block.

placing the left-sided needle first, a single needle can often be used for the block. If the aorta is penetrated en route, a transaortic technique is employed. A 22-gauge, 5-inch spinal needle (8 inches for the obese patient) is advanced just caudal to the margin of the twelfth rib and cephalad to the transverse process of L1 toward the anterolateral surface of the L1 vertebral body. The needle is advanced, using repeat images every 1 to 2 cm of advancement to ensure the needle remains coaxial until the needle contacts the anterolateral margin of L1. The c-arm is then rotated to a lateral projection, and the needle is advanced to lie 2 to 3 cm anterior to the anterior margin of L1 in the lateral view (Fig. 11-4). Continuous aspiration should be applied as the needle is advanced anterior to the anterior border of L1. If blood appears, the needle has penetrated the aorta and should be advanced through the anterior wall of the aorta, until blood can no longer be aspirated. The needle tip should be medial to the lateral border of the L1 vertebral body in the AP view (Fig. 11-5). Final needle position is confirmed by injecting 1 to 2 mL of radiographic contrast (iohexol 180 mg per mL) under live fluoroscopy. The contrast should layer over the anterior surface of the aorta (see Fig. 11-4) and appear pulsatile. If the contrast spreads to both sides of midline over the anterior surface of the aorta (Fig. 11-6), then only a single needle is necessary for the block. If the contrast remains to the left of midline over the anterolateral surface of the aorta, a second

needle is placed from the contralateral side using the same technique described for the left-sided block. The final needle location for celiac plexus block and the adjacent structures are illustrated in Figure 11-7. Diagnostic celiac plexus block prior to neurolysis is carried out using 20 to 30 mL of 0.25% bupivacaine (10 to 15 mL per side). The dose should be given in increments of 5 mL, aspirating periodically to ensure the needle has not moved to an intravascular location.

Splanchnic Nerve Block (Retrocrural Technique)

Once the c-arm is aligned, the skin and subcutaneous tissues overlying the anterolateral margin of the midportion of the T12 vertebral body are anesthetized with 1 to 2 mL of 1% lidocaine. For splanchnic nerve block and neurolysis, needles must be placed on both sides. A 22-gauge, 5-inch spinal needle (8 inches for the obese patient) is advanced just caudal to the margin of the twelfth rib and cephalad to the transverse process of L1 toward the anterolateral surface of the T12 vertebral body. This requires 20 to 30 degrees of cephalad angulation of the c-arm (see Figs. 11-1 and 11-2). The needle is advanced, using repeat images every 1 to 2 cm of advancement to ensure the needle remains coaxial until the needle contacts the anterolateral margin of T12. The c-arm is then rotated to a lateral projection, and the needle is advanced 1 to 2 cm to align with the anterior one-third of the

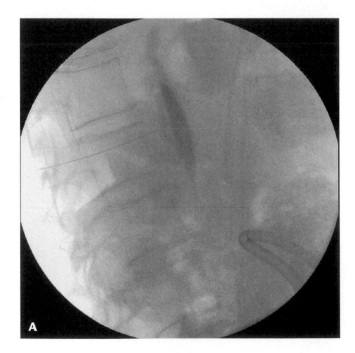 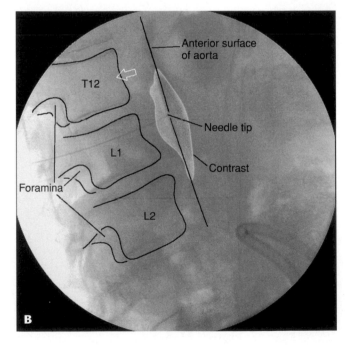

Figure 11-4.
Lateral radiograph of the spine during celiac plexus block. **A:** A single needle is in final position over the anterolateral surface of the aorta, approximately 2 cm anterior to the vertebral body of L1. Radiographic contrast (2 mL of iohexol 180 mg per mL) has been injected. The contrast layers over the anterior surface of the aorta and during live fluoroscopy, pulsation of the aorta can be seen. Note the slight rotation of the vertebral bodies such that the left and right intervertebral foramina are not aligned. **B:** Labeled image. The white arrow indicates the final needle position for splanchnic nerve block.

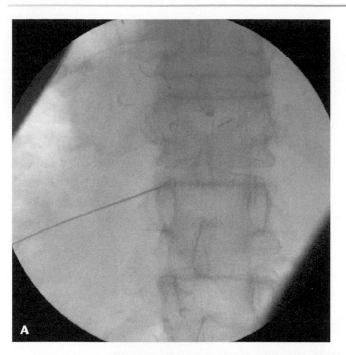
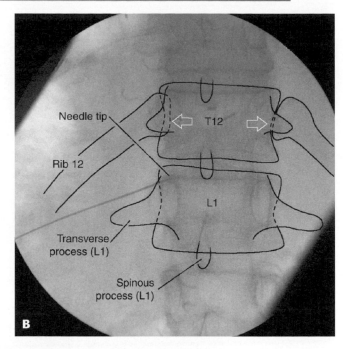

Figure 11-5.
Anterior-Posterior radiograph of the spine during celiac plexus block. **A:** A single needle has been inserted from a left oblique approach and is in final position over the anterolateral surface of the aorta. **B:** Labeled image. The white arrows indicate the final needle position for splanchnic nerve block.

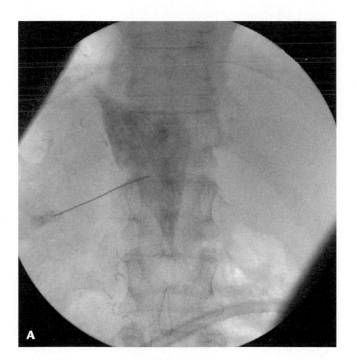
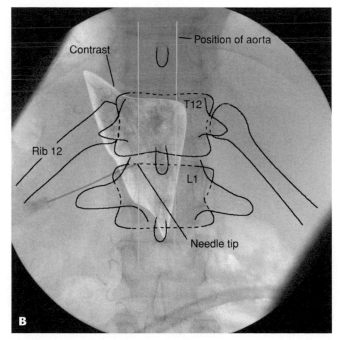

Figure 11-6.
Anterior-Posterior radiograph of the spine during celiac plexus block. **A:** A single needle has been inserted from a left oblique approach and is in final position over the anterolateral surface of the aorta. Radiographic contrast (2 mL of iohexol 180 mg per mL) has been injected followed by 20 mL of 0.25% bupivacaine. The local anesthetic has diluted the contrast and extended the spread. A portion of the contrast spreads along the inferior border of the left hemidiaphragm. **B:** Labeled image. The approximate position of the aorta is shown.

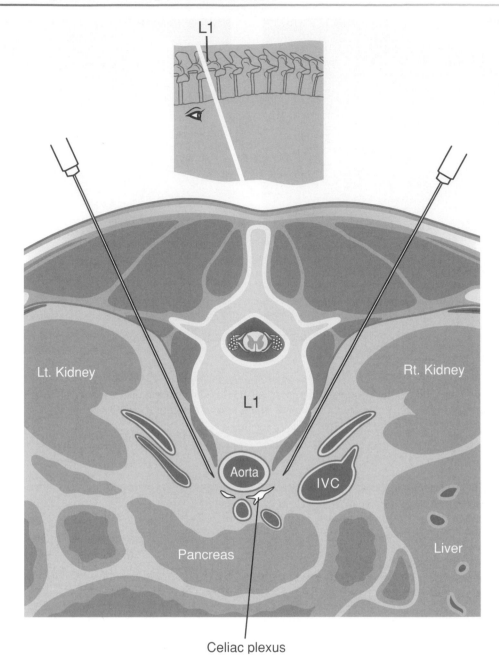

Figure 11-7.
Axial diagram of celiac plexus block. Two needles pass through the crura of the diaphragm adjacent to the L1 vertebral body and are in final position over the anterolateral surface of the aorta. The inset indicates the approximate plane of the needles.

T12 vertebral body in the lateral view (see Fig. 11-4). The needle tip should be just medial to the lateral border of the T12 vertebral body in the anterior-posterior view (see Fig. 11-5). Final needle position is confirmed by injecting 1 to 2 mL of radiographic contrast (iohexol 180 mg per mL) under live fluoroscopy. The contrast should layer over the antero-lateral surface of the T12 vertebral body. A second needle is placed from the contralateral side, using the same technique described for the left-sided block. The final needle location for splanchnic nerve block and the adjacent structures are

illustrated in Figure 11-8. Diagnostic splanchnic nerve block prior to neurolysis is carried out using 10 to 15 mL 0.25% bupivacaine (5 to 8 mL per side). The dose should be given in increments of 5 mL or less, aspirating periodically to ensure the needle has not moved to an intravascular location.

Celiac Plexus and Splanchnic Neurolysis

The technique for needle placement is identical for diagnostic local anesthetic block of the celiac plexus or splanchnic

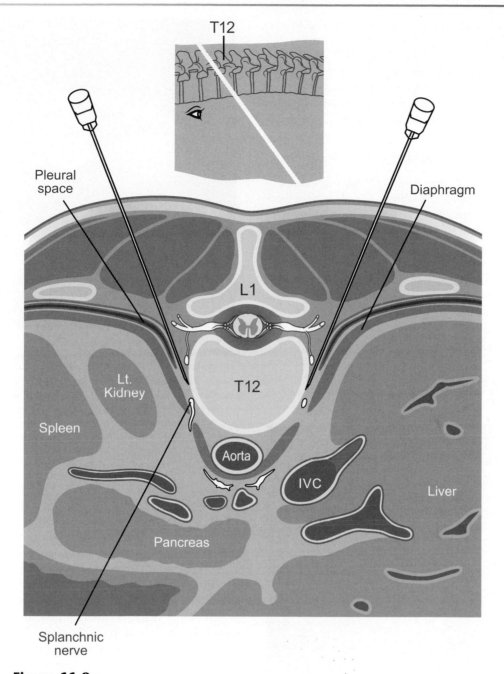

Figure 11-8.
Axial diagram of splanchnic nerve block. Two needles remain posterior to the crura of the diaphragm and are in final position over the anterolateral surface of the T12 vertebral body. The inset indicates the approximate plane of the needles.

nerves and for neurolysis. The two commonly used neurolytic solutions are ethyl alcohol and phenol. The pharmacology of these agents is discussed in detail in Chapter 4. A 10% to 12% solution of phenol can be prepared in radiographic contrast (iohexol 180 mg per mL). This allows the spread of the neurolytic solution to be monitored radiographically as it is injected. For celiac plexus neurolysis, 20 to 30 mL (10 to 15 mL per side) is injected. If the neurolytic solution spreads to both sides of midline over the anterior surface of the aorta (see Fig. 11-6), then only a single needle

is necessary for the block. If the neurolytic solution begins to spread posteriorly toward the intervertebral foramen, the injection should be halted to avoid nerve root injury. During splanchnic neurolysis, the contrast should layer over the anterolateral surface of the T12 vertebral body. A second needle is placed from the contralateral side using the same technique described for the left-sided block. For splanchnic neurolysis, 10 to 15 mL (5 to 8 mL per side) is injected. The needles should be flushed with saline or local anesthetic before they are removed to avoid depositing the neurolytic solution along the needle track. Neurolysis can also be carried out using 50% to 100% ethyl alcohol in similar volumes. Phenol has a direct local anesthetic effect and is associated with minimal pain on injection. Ethyl alcohol produces intense burning pain on injection and is best diluted with local anesthetic prior to injection or injected after placing a small volume of local anesthetic.

Computed Tomography-guided Celiac Plexus Block

Although the majority of cases can be carried out using fluoroscopic guidance alone, CT allows excellent visualization of the anatomic structures that lie in close proximity to the target site during NCPB. To directly ablate the celiac plexus, the needles must be advanced through the diaphragm until they lie adjacent to the anterolateral surface of the aorta. This can be accomplished by advancing two separate needles adjacent to the anterolateral surface of the aorta (Fig. 11-9) or using a single needle advanced through the aorta (Fig. 11-10). CT allows visualization of the structures that lie adjacent to the celiac ganglion.

CT-guided celiac plexus block is carried out with the patient positioned prone in the CT scanner gantry with the head turned to one side (Fig. 11-11). A radiographic marker

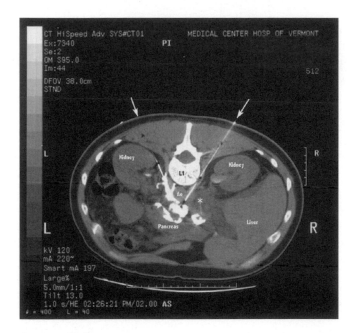

Figure 11-9.
Computed tomography after placement of two transcrural needles for neurolytic celiac plexus block. Neurolytic solution (10% phenol in iohexol 100 mg per mL) has been injected through both needles (10 mL on each side). The arrows indicate the approximate needle trajectory on each side. Contrast extends over the left anterolateral surface of the aorta and anteriorly along the posterior surface of the pancreas. There is a large soft-tissue mass adjacent to the right-sided needle (*asterisk*) consistent with adenopathy or metastatic tumor. (Reprinted from Rathmell JP, Gallant JM, Brown DL. Computed tomography and the anatomy of celiac plexus block. *Reg Anesth Pain Med.* 2000;25:412, with permission.)

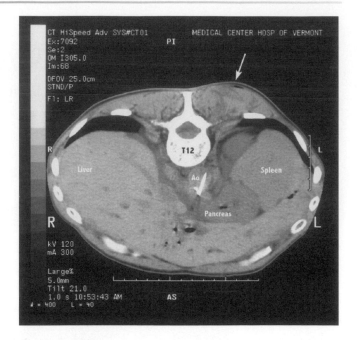

Figure 11-10.
Computed tomography after placement of a single transaortic needle. The arrow indicates the approximate trajectory of the needle. The medial pleural reflection can be seen passing within 2 mm of the needle's path. (Reprinted from Rathmell JP, Gallant JM, Brown DL. Computed tomography and the anatomy of celiac plexus block. *Reg Anesth Pain Med.* 2000;25: 414, with permission.)

is placed on the skin surface 1 cm inferior to the inferior margin of the twelfth rib and 7 cm from midline, and axial CT images extending from T12 through L1 are taken in 3-mm intervals. In this way, the position of the needle entry site on the skin's surface can be adjusted to form a direct path to the anterolateral surface of the aorta, without passing through adjacent structures (see Fig. 11-9). The skin is anesthetized with 1 to 2 mL of 1% lidocaine, and a 22-gauge, 5-inch spinal needle is then seated in a plane that corresponds to the axis seen on CT (the exact angle can be calculated using software available within the CT scanner). With the needle seated in the subcutaneous tissue, but still superficial, a repeat CT image is obtained through the tip of the needle (Fig. 11-12A), and the angle of the needle is then redirected toward the anterolateral surface of the aorta (Fig. 11-12B). The needle is advanced and repeat CT images are obtained after every 1 to 2 cm of needle advancement. Once the needle is in position, a small volume of radiographic contrast is injected to confirm needle position (0.5 mL of iohexol 100 mg per mL is sufficient). A 10% to 12% solution of phenol in radiographic contrast (iohexol 100 mg per mL) allows the spread of the neurolytic solution to be monitored radiographically as it is injected. A repeat CT image is obtained after every 5 mL of injection. For celiac plexus neurolysis, 20 to 30 mL (10 to 15 mL per side) is injected. If the neurolytic solution spreads to both sides of midline over the anterior surface of the aorta, then only a single needle is necessary for the block.

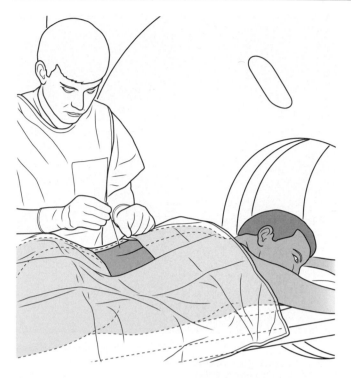

Figure 11-11.
Patient position for computed tomography (CT)-guided celiac plexus block. The patient is placed prone in the CT scanner gantry with the arms overhead and the head turned to one side. The operator stands to one side and advances the needle using a position and trajectory determined via the CT axial images (see Fig. 11-12).

Complications

There are several physiologic side effects that are expected following celiac plexus block. These include diarrhea and orthostatic hypotension. Blockade of the sympathetic innervation to the abdominal viscera results in unopposed parasympathetic innervation of the alimentary tract, and may produce abdominal cramping and sudden diarrhea. Likewise, the vasodilation that ensues often results in orthostatic hypotension. These effects are invariably transient but may persist for several days after neurolytic block. The hypotension seldom requires treatment other than intravenous hydration.

Complications of celiac plexus and splanchnic nerve block include hematuria, intravascular injection, and pneumothorax. CT allows visualization of the structures that lie adjacent to the celiac ganglion as the block is being performed (see Figs. 11-9 and 11-10). The kidneys extend between T12 and L3, with the left kidney slightly more cephalad than the right. The aorta lies over the left anterolateral border of the vertebral column. The celiac arterial trunk arises from the anterior surface of the aorta at the T12 level and divides into the hepatic, left gastric, and splenic arteries. Using the transaortic technique, caution must be used to avoid needle placement directly through the axis of the celiac trunk as it exits anteriorly. The inferior vena cava lies just to the right of the aorta over the anterolateral surface of the vertebral column. The medial pleural reflection extends inferomedially as low as the T12 to L1 level.

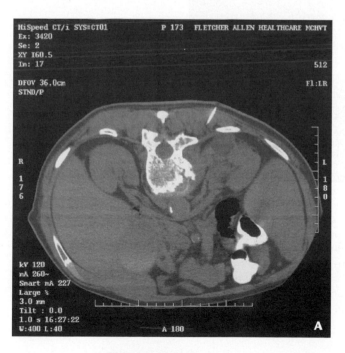

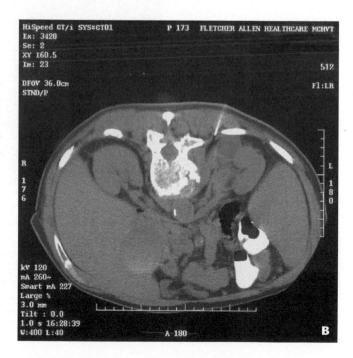

Figure 11-12.
Sequential axial images during computed tomography-guided celiac plexus block.
A: Axial image at the L1 vertebral level with the needle seated just beneath the skin. Note the needle is aimed directly at the transverse process. **B:** The needle direction has been corrected to pass lateral to the transverse process and toward the anterolateral surface of the aorta.

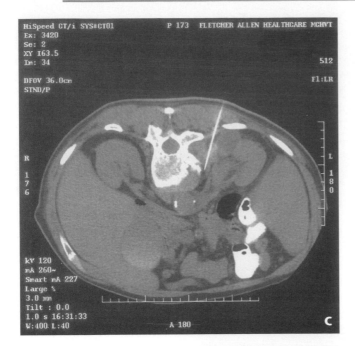

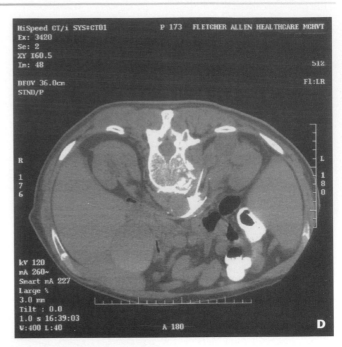

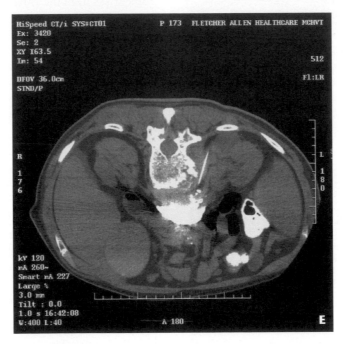

Figure 11-12. *(Continued)*
C: Repeat axial images are obtained after every 1 to 2 cm of needle advancement and here shows the needle passing lateral to the L1 vertebral body. **D:** Axial image with the needle in final position over the anterolateral surface of the aorta and showing good spread of contrast over the anterior surface of the aorta (1 mL of iohexol 100 mg per mL). **E:** Final axial image after placement of 15 mL of 10% phenol in iohexol 100 mg per mL. The contrast spreads over the entire anterior surface of the aorta without extending to the posterior surface of the aorta or the intervertebral foramina. Placement of a second needle on the contralateral side is not needed.

NCPB carries small but significant additional risk. Intravascular injection of 30 mL of 100% ethanol will result in a blood ethanol level well above the legal limit for intoxication but below danger of severe alcohol toxicity. Intravascular injection of phenol is associated with clinical manifestations similar to that of local anesthetic toxicity—central nervous system excitation, followed by seizures, and in extreme toxicity, cardiovascular collapse. The most devastating complication associated with NCPB using either alcohol or phenol is paraplegia. The theoretical mechanism is spread of the neurolytic solution toward the posterior surface of the aorta to surround the spinal segmental arteries. At the level of T12 or L1, it is common to have a single, dominant spinal segmental artery, the artery of Adamkiewicz. In some individuals, this artery is the dominant arterial supply to the anterior two-thirds of the spinal cord in the low thoracic region. Neurolytic solution may cause spasm or even necrosis and occlusion of the artery of Adamkiewicz leading to paralysis. The actual incidence of this complication is unknown, but it appears to be less than 1:1,000.

SUGGESTED READINGS

Bridenbaugh LD, Moore DC, Campbell DD. Management of upper abdominal cancer pain: treatment with celiac plexus block with alcohol. *JAMA.* 1964;190:877–880.

Brown DL. *Atlas of Regional Anesthesia.* 2nd ed. Philadelphia: WB Saunders; 1999:281–292.

Eisenberg E, Carr DB, Chalmers TC. Neurolytic celiac plexus block for treatment of cancer pain: a meta-analysis. *Anesth Analg.* 1995;80:290–295.

Ischia S, Polati E, Finco G et al. 1998 Labat lecture: the role of the neurolytic celiac plexus block in pancreatic cancer pain management: do we have the answers? *Reg Anesth Pain Med.* 1998;23:611–614.

Lamer TJ. Sympathetic nerve blocks. In: Brown DL, ed. *Regional Anesthesia and Analgesia.* Philadelphia: WB Saunders; 1996:357–384.

Lieberman RP, Waldman SD. Celiac plexus neurolysis with the modified transaortic approach. *Radiology.* 1990;175:274–276.

Rathmell JP. Sympathetic blocks. In: Rathmell JP, Neal JM, Viscomi CV, eds. *Requisites in Anesthesiology: Regional Anesthesia.* Philadelphia: Elsevier Health Sciences; 2004:128–141.

Rathmell JP, Gallant JM, Brown DL. Computed tomography and the anatomy of celiac plexus block. *Reg Anesth Pain Med.* 2000;25:411–416.

Rauck R. Sympathetic nerve blocks: head, neck, and trunk. In: Raj PP, ed. *Practical Management of Pain.* 3rd ed. St. Louis, MO: Mosby; 2000: 651–682.

Lumbar Sympathetic Block and Neurolysis

Overview

The sympathetic nervous system is involved in the pathophysiology that leads to a number of different chronic pain conditions, including complex regional pain syndrome (CRPS) and ischemic pain. These chronic pain states are often referred to as *sympathetically maintained pain* because they share the characteristic of pain relief following blockade of the regional sympathetic ganglia. Lumbar sympathetic block is an established method for the diagnosis and treatment of sympathetically maintained pain of the lower extremities.

Anatomy

The lumbar sympathetic chain consists of four to five paired ganglia that lie over the anterolateral surface of the second through fourth lumbar vertebrae (Figs. 12-1 and 12-2). The cell bodies that travel to the lumbar sympathetic ganglia lie in the anterolateral region of the spinal cord from T11 to L2, with variable contributions from T10 and L3. The preganglionic fibers leave the spinal canal with the corresponding spinal nerve root, join the sympathetic chain as white communicating rami, and then synapse within the appropriate ganglion. Postganglionic fibers exit the chain to join the diffuse perivascular plexus around the iliac and femoral arteries, or via the gray communicating rami to join the nerve roots that form the lumbar and lumbosacral plexuses. Sympathetic fibers accompany all the major nerves to the lower extremities. The majority of the sympathetic innervation to the lower extremities passes through the second and

third lumbar sympathetic ganglia, and blockade of these ganglia results in near complete sympathetic denervation of the lower extremities.

Patient Selection

Lumbar sympathetic blockade has been used extensively in the treatment of sympathetically maintained pain syndromes involving the lower extremities. The most common of these are CRPS, type 1 (reflex sympathetic dystrophy) and type 2 (causalgia) (see Chapter 10 for an overview of CRPS). The local anesthetic block can produce marked pain relief of long duration, and this block is used as part of a comprehensive treatment plan to provide analgesia and facilitate functional restoration.

Patients with peripheral vascular insufficiency due to small vessel occlusion may also be treated effectively with lumbar sympathetic blockade. Proximal fixed lesions are best treated with surgical intervention using bypass grafting or intra-arterial stent placement to restore blood flow. In those patients with diffuse, small vessel occlusion, lumbar sympathetic block can improve microvascular circulation and reduce ischemic pain. If local anesthetic block improves blood flow and reduces pain, these patients will often benefit from surgical or chemical sympathectomy.

Other patients with neuropathic pain involving the lower extremities have shown variable response to lumbar sympathetic block. In those with acute herpes zoster and early postherpetic neuralgia, sympathetic block may reduce pain. However, once postherpetic neuralgia is well established (beyond 3 to 6 months from onset), sympathetic blockade is rarely helpful. Likewise, deafferentation syndromes such as phantom limb pain and neuropathic lower-extremity pain following spinal cord injury have shown variable and largely disappointing responses to sympathetic blockade.

Positioning

The patient lies prone with the head turned to one side (Fig. 12-3). The c-arm is centered over the midlumbar region. The final needle position for lumbar sympathetic block is over the anterolateral surface of the lumbar vertebral body (see Fig. 12-2). The c-arm is rotated obliquely 20 to 30

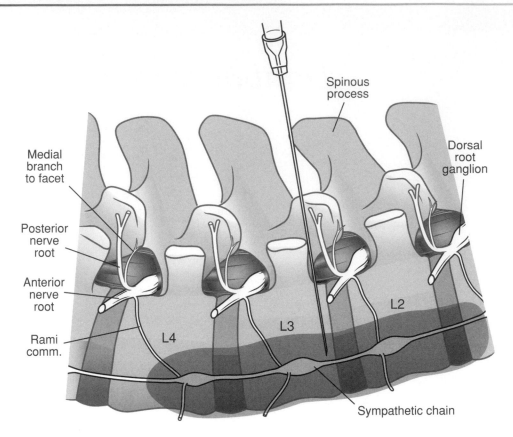

Figure 12-1.
Anatomy of the lumbar sympathetic chain. The lumbar sympathetic ganglia are variable in number and location from one individual to another. Most commonly, the ganglia lie over the anteromedial surface of the vertebral bodies between L2 and L4. Temporary lumbar sympathetic block using local anesthetic is best performed by advancing a single needle cephalad to the transverse process of L3 to avoid the exiting nerve root. The needle tip is placed adjacent to the superior portion of the anteromedial surface of the L3 vertebral body. Use of 15 to 20 mL of local anesthetic solution will spread to cover multiple vertebral levels (*shaded region*).

degrees, until the tip of the transverse process of L3 overlies the anterolateral margin of the L3 vertebral body (Fig. 12-4).

Block Technique

Lumbar sympathetic block is typically carried out using a single needle technique and using a large volume of local anesthetic to spread cephalad and caudad to bathe adjacent ganglia. The ganglia of the lumbar sympathetic chain are variable in number and location from one individual to another. The ganglia lie between L2 and L4, and in most humans the ganglia lie over the inferior portion of L2 and the superior portion of L3. Thus, the optimal location to place a single needle is over the anterolateral margin of the inferior portion of L2, the L2/L3 interspace, or the superior margin of L3.

The patient is placed in the prone position with a pillow under the lower abdomen and iliac crest to reduce the lumbar lordosis (see Fig. 12-3). The skin and subcutaneous tissues are anesthetized with 1 to 2 mL of 1% lidocaine. A 22-gauge, 5-inch spinal needle (7 to 8 inches for obese

patients) is advanced using a coaxial technique toward the anterolateral surface of the L3 vertebral body (see Fig. 12-4). The direction of the needle is assessed and redirected by obtaining repeat images after every 1 to 1.5 cm of needle advancement. The needle tip should be kept over the lateral margin of the vertebral body until the needle gently contacts bone. An additional 1 to 1.5 mL of 1% lidocaine is placed on the vertebral body, and the needle is then walked laterally off the bony margin. The c-arm is rotated to a lateral projection, and the needle is advanced until the tip lies over the anterior one-third of the vertebral body (Fig. 12-5). Proper needle position is verified in the anterior-posterior (AP) projection, where the needle tip should lie medial to the lateral margin of the vertebral body (Fig. 12-6).

Once the needle is in position, aspiration to detect intravascular needle placement is carried out, followed by the incremental injection of local anesthetic (15 to 20 mL of 0.25% bupivacaine). Signs of successful sympathetic blockade in the lower extremities include venodilation and temperature rise. The skin temperature should also be

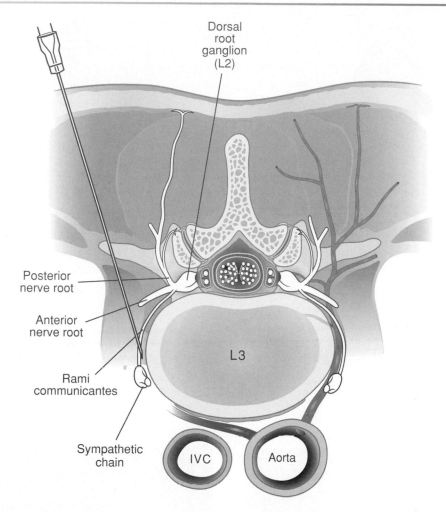

Figure 12-2.
Axial diagram of lumbar sympathetic block. A single needle passes over the transverse process, and the tip is in position adjacent to the lumbar sympathetic ganglia over the anteromedial surface of the L3 vertebral body.

monitored in the contralateral foot to assess for changes unrelated to the block. A rise in temperature of at least 1°C without a rise in the temperature of the contralateral limb should occur with successful sympathetic block.

Lumbar Sympathetic Neurolysis

Neurolytic lumbar sympathetic block has been used in efforts to provide long-term sympathetic blockade in those who receive only short-term pain relief with local anesthetic blocks. Lumbar sympathetic neurolysis can be accomplished using either injection of a neurolytic solution or radiofrequency lesioning. Because the locations of the lumbar sympathetic ganglia are variable, injection of neurolytic solution that spreads to encompass an area beyond the needle tip may produce more reliable neurolysis than radiofrequency treatment. Nonetheless, when the needle tips are positioned accurately, the discrete lesions resulting from radiofrequency treatment can produce effective neurolysis. Although the

techniques are well described, there are few data available to guide the choice among chemical neurolysis, radiofrequency neurolysis, and open surgical sympathectomy.

Chemical Neurolysis

Chemical neurolysis of the lumbar sympathetic chain is carried out by placing three separate needles at the L2, L3, and L4 levels as described previously for local anesthetic block (Figs. 12-7 and 12-8). The needles should be directed to the mid- or inferior aspect of L2, as well as the superior aspects of L3 and L4, to correlate with the most frequent anatomic locations of the lumbar sympathetic ganglia. Three needles are placed so that the smallest volume of neurolytic solution can be injected to treat the ganglia at each level. Once proper needle position has been confirmed in the AP and lateral projections, a small volume of radiographic contrast (1 mL of iohexol 180 mg per mL) is placed through each needle to ensure the needles are not

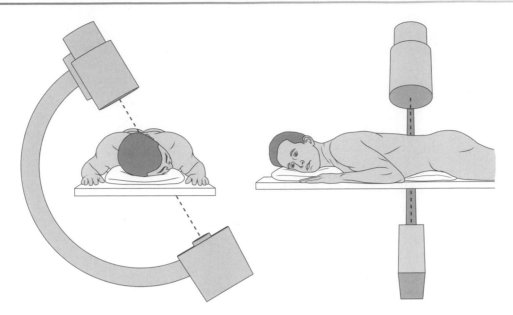

Figure 12-3.
Patient position for lumbar sympathetic block. The patient lies prone with the head turned to one side. The c-arm is positioned over the midlumbar spine with 20 to 30 degrees of oblique angulation.

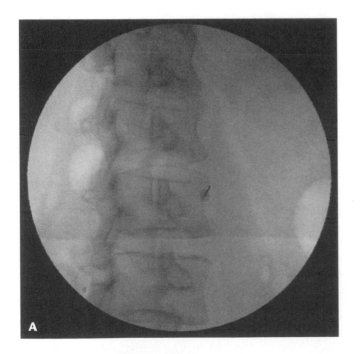
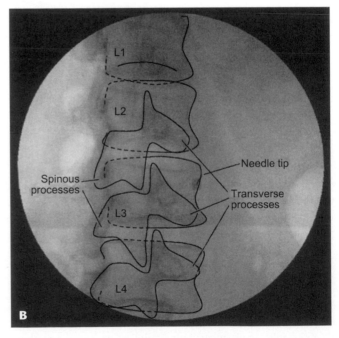

Figure 12-4.
Oblique radiograph of the lumbar spine during lumbar sympathetic block. **A:** A needle passes cephalad to the transverse process of L3 to lie anterolateral to the superior aspect of the L3 vertebral body. **B:** Labeled image.

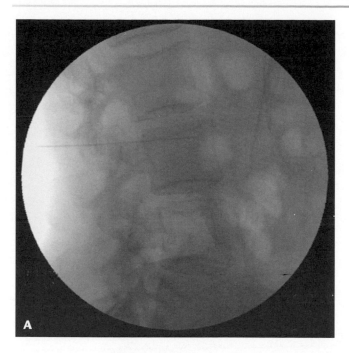
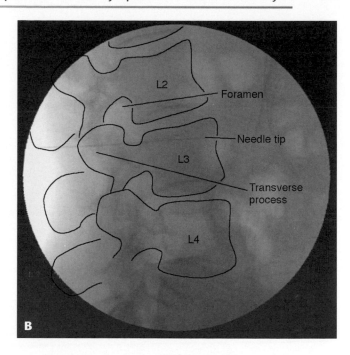

Figure 12-5.
Lateral radiograph of the lumbar spine during lumbar sympathetic block. **A:** A needle is in position over the anterolateral surface of L3. The tip should be positioned over the anterior one-third of the vertebral body in the lateral projection. Note that the foramen, and thus the exiting nerve root, are distant from the path of the needle. **B:** Labeled image.

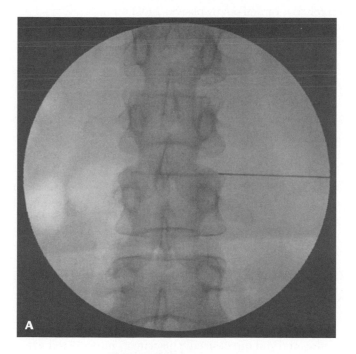
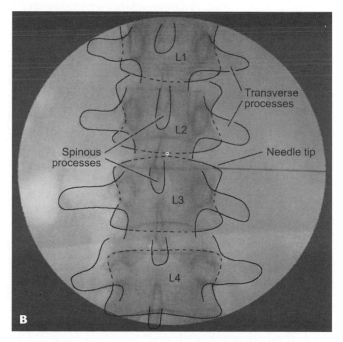

Figure 12-6.
Anterior-Posterior (AP) radiograph of the lumbar spine during lumbar sympathetic block. **A:** A needle passes cephalad to the transverse process of L3, and the tip lies over the anterolateral surface of L3. When positioned correctly, the needle tip should lie medial to the lateral margin of the vertebral body in the AP projection. This indicates that the tip of the needle is in close apposition to the anterolateral surface of the vertebral body. **B:** Labeled image.

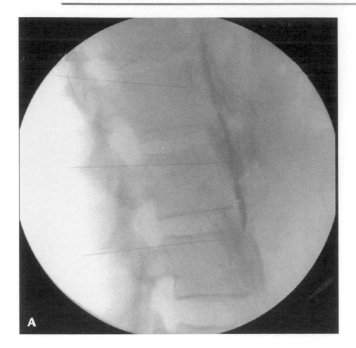

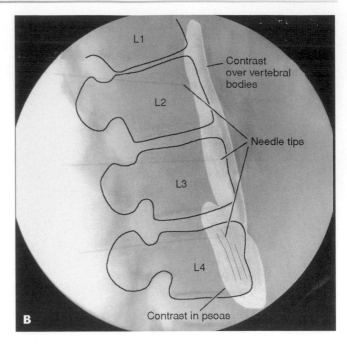

Figure 12-7.
Lateral radiograph of the lumbar spine during neurolytic lumbar sympathetic block.
A: Three needles are in position with their tips over the anterolateral surface of L2, L3, and L4. One milliliter of radiographic contrast (iohexol 180 mg per mL) has been placed through each needle. Contrast has spread tightly adjacent to the anterolateral surface of the vertebral bodies through the needles at L2 and L3. The contrast adjacent to the needle at L4 has spread more diffusely in an anterior and inferior direction, indicating injection within the psoas muscle (see also Fig. 12-8). This needle must be repositioned before neurolysis in a more anterior and medial direction. Neurolysis is carried out by placing 2 to 3 mL of neurolytic solution (10% phenol in iohexol 180 mg per mL or 50% to 100% ethyl alcohol) through each needle. The needle position for radiofrequency neurolysis is identical.
B: Labeled image.

intravascular and the injectate will layer in close apposition to the anterolateral margin of the vertebral bodies (see Figs. 12-7 and 12-8). Thereafter, 2 to 3 mL of neurolytic solution (10% phenol in iohexol 180 mg per mL or 50 to 100% ethyl alcohol) are placed through each needle.

Radiofrequency Neurolysis

Similar to chemical neurolysis, radiofrequency neurolysis of the lumbar sympathetic chain is carried out by placing three separate 15-cm radiofrequency cannulae with 10-mm active tips over the anterolateral surface of the L2, L3, and L4 vertebral bodies (see Figs. 12-7 and 12-8). Once proper needle position has been confirmed, sensory and motor stimulation are conducted. When the cannulae are in proper position over the sympathetic ganglia, the patient will typically report vague back or abdominal discomfort with less than 1 V of output with sensory stimulation at 50 Hz. However, the report of any sensation during sensory testing is more variable than during sensory testing before radiofrequency treatment of the facets. Motor stimulation is then carried out to ensure the can-

nulae do not lie along the course of the anterior primary ramus of one of the spinal nerve roots. There should be no muscle movement in the lower extremities during stimulation at 2 Hz at an output of at least 3 V. Our practice has been to place the lesions if the cannulae appear to be in the proper anatomic position, even if there is no report of pain or discomfort during sensory stimulation. Lesions are created after instilling 0.5 mL of 2% lidocaine at 80°C for 90 seconds.

▓▓▓ Complications

Significant and potentially toxic levels of local anesthetic can result from direct needle placement into a blood vessel and intravascular injection during lumbar sympathetic block. Hematuria can follow direct needle placement through the kidney and is usually self-limited. Nerve root, epidural, or intrathecal injection can arise when the needle is advanced through the intervertebral foramen and is usually avoided entirely with proper use of radiographic guidance. Following neurolytic lumbar sympathetic block,

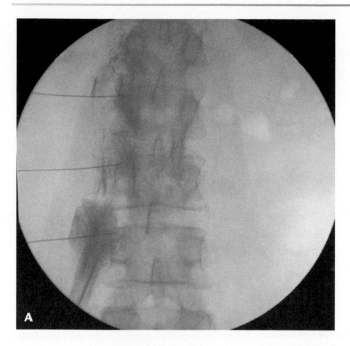

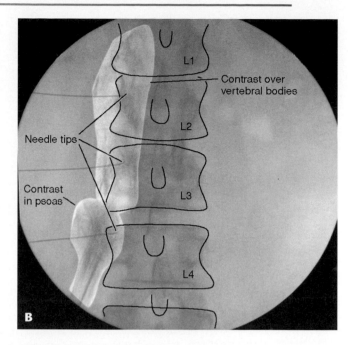

Figure 12-8.

Anterior-Posterior radiograph of the lumbar spine during neurolytic lumbar sympathetic block. **A:** Three needles are in position with their tips over the anterolateral surface of L2, L3, and L4. One milliliter of radiographic contrast (iohexol 180 mg per mL) has been placed through each needle. Contrast has spread tightly adjacent to the anterolateral surface of the vertebral bodies through the needles at L2 and L3. The contrast adjacent to the needle at L4 has spread more diffusely in a lateral and inferior direction, indicating injection within the psoas muscle (see also Fig. 12-7). This needle must be repositioned before neurolysis in a more anterior and medial direction. Neurolysis is carried out by placing 2 to 3 mL of neurolytic solution (10% phenol in iohexol 180 mg per mL or 50% to 100% ethyl alcohol) through each needle. The needle position for radiofrequency neurolysis is identical. **B:** Labeled image.

significant postsympathectomy pain arises in the L1 and L2 nerve root distribution over the anterior thigh in as many as 10% of treated patients. This observation stems from the results following open surgical sympathectomy, but such postsympathectomy neuralgia has also been reported after both chemical and radiofrequency sympathectomy. Postsympathectomy neuralgic pain in the anterior thigh has been postulated to result from partial neurolysis of adjacent sensory fibers, most often the genitofemoral nerve.

SUGGESTED READINGS

Breivik H, Cousins MJ, Löfström JB. Sympathetic neural blockade of upper and lower extremity. In: Cousins MJ, Bridenbaugh PO, eds. *Neural Blockade in Clinical Anesthesia and Management of Pain.* 3rd ed. Philadelphia: Lippincott-Raven; 1998:411–447.

Brown DL. *Atlas of Regional Anesthesia.* 2nd ed. Philadelphia: WB Saunders; 1999:275–279.

Cousins MJ, Reeve TS, Glynn CJ et al. Neurolytic lumbar sympathetic blockade: duration of denervation and relief of rest pain. *Anaesth Intensive Care.* 1979;7:121–135.

Lamer TJ. Sympathetic nerve blocks. In: Brown DL, ed. *Regional Anesthesia and Analgesia.* Philadelphia: WB Saunders; 1996:357–384.

Rathmell JP. Sympathetic blocks. In: Rathmell JP, Neal JM, Viscomi CV, eds. *Requisites in Anesthesiology: Regional Anesthesia.* Philadelphia: Elsevier Health Sciences; 2004:128–141.

Rocco AG. Radiofrequency lumbar sympatholysis. The evolution of a technique for managing sympathetically maintained pain. *Reg Anesth.* 1995;20:3–12.

Rocco AG, Palombi D, Raeke D. Anatomy of the lumbar sympathetic chain. *Reg Anesth.* 1995;20:13–19.

Superior Hypogastric Block and Neurolysis

Overview

The sympathetic nervous system is involved in the pathophysiology that leads to a number of different chronic pain conditions, including pain arising from the bladder, uterus, rectum, vagina, and prostate. The relevant anatomy and technique for superior hypogastric block has been well described, but only limited observational data point to the usefulness of this technique for treating chronic pain arising from the pelvic viscera.

Anatomy

The superior hypogastric plexus is composed of a flattened band of intercommunicating nerve fibers that descend over the aortic bifurcation. The plexus carries sympathetic afferents and postganglionic efferent fibers from the lumbar sympathetic chain, as well parasympathetic fibers that arise from S2 to S4. The plexus is retroperitoneal in location and lies over the anterior surface of the fourth and fifth lumbar and the first sacral vertebrae (Figs. 13-1 and 13-2). Sympathetic nerves passing through the plexus innervate the pelvic viscera, including the bladder, uterus, rectum, vagina, and prostate.

Patient Selection

Superior hypogastric plexus block is used in the treatment of pain arising from the pelvic viscera. In patients with pain of nonmalignant origin, temporary block may be useful in better defining the source of the pain. More often, superior hypogastric neurolysis is used to treat intractable pelvic visceral pain associated with malignancy. Patients with locally invasive cancer involving the proximal vagina, uterus, ovaries, prostate and rectum that are associated with pelvic pain often gain significant pain relief from this approach.

Positioning

The patient and c-arm positioning for superior hypogastric block are similar to those used for discography at the L5/S1 level (Fig. 13-3). The target for needle placement lies over the anterolateral surface of the L5/S1 junction (see Fig. 13-2). The patient lies prone, with the head turned to one side. A pillow is placed under the lower abdomen, above the iliac crest, in an effort to reduce the lumbar lordosis. Asking the patient to rotate the inferior aspect of the pelvis anteriorly toward the table will tip the iliac crests posteriorly and is often key to successfully performing this block. The c-arm is rotated 25 to 35 degrees obliquely and centered on the lumbosacral junction. The c-arm is then angled with 25 to 35 degrees of cephalad angulation, and the L5/S1 disc is brought into view.

Block Technique

With the c-arm properly aligned, there is a small triangular window through which the needle must pass to reach the anterolateral margin of the lumbosacral junction. The triangle is bounded superiorly by the transverse process of L5, laterally by the iliac crest, and medially by the L5/S1 facet joint, structures that are readily identified using fluoroscopy (Fig. 13-4). A skin entry point is made over the lowest point of this triangle and typically overlies the iliac crest, 5 to 7 cm from midline at the level of the L5 spinous process. A 22-gauge, 5-inch needle (8 inches for obese patients) is advanced using fluoroscopic guidance to lie anterolateral to the L5/S1 intervertebral disc or the inferior margin of the L5 vertebral body (Figs. 13-5 and 13-6). A small volume (2 to 3 mL) of radiographic contrast material will spread along the anterior surface of the lumbosacral junction, confirming correct needle position (Figs. 13-7 and 13-8). The same procedure is then carried out on the contralateral side. Temporary block is performed with 8 to 10 mL of local anesthetic (0.25% bupivacaine).

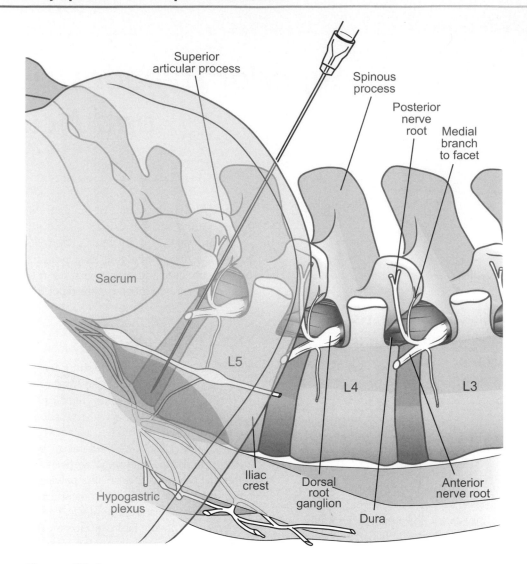

Figure 13-1.

Anatomy of the superior hypogastric plexus. The superior hypogastric plexus is comprised of a loose, weblike group of interlacing nerve fibers that lie over the anterolateral surface of the L5 vertebral body and extend inferiorly over the sacrum. Needles are positioned over the anterolateral surface of the L5/S1 intervertebral disc or the inferior aspect of the L5 vertebral bodies to block the superior hypogastric plexus. Use of 8 to 10 mL of local anesthetic solution will spread along the anterior surface of the L5 vertebral body and the sacrum *(shaded area)*.

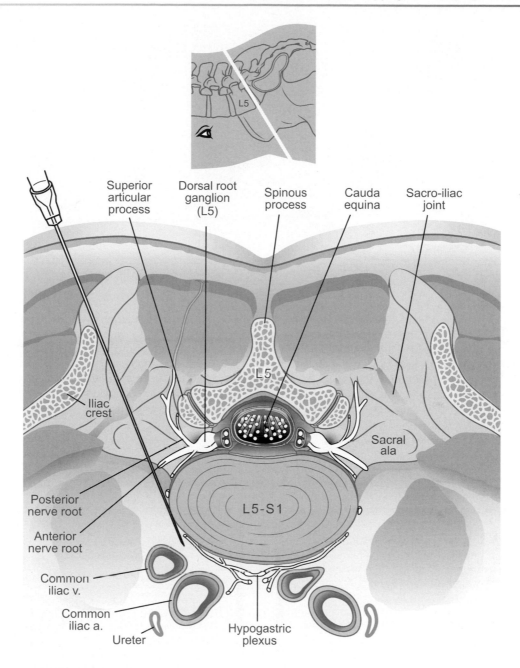

Figure 13-2.

Axial diagram of superior hypogastric plexus block. Needles are advanced from either side over the junction between the sacral ala and the superior articular process of S1 to position the needle tips over the anterolateral surface of the L5/S1 disc space. Note the close proximity of the iliac vessels. The inset shows the plane and orientation of the axial diagram.

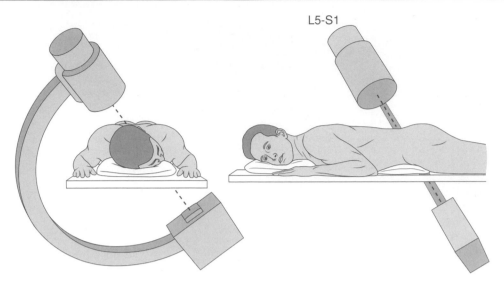

L5-S1

Figure 13-3.
Patient position for superior hypogastric plexus block. The patient lies prone, with the head turned to one side. A pillow is placed under the lower abdomen, above the iliac crest, in an effort to reduce the lumbar lordosis. Asking the patient to rotate the inferior aspect of the pelvis anteriorly toward the table will tip the iliac crests posteriorly and is often key to successfully performing this block. The c-arm is rotated 25 to 35 degrees obliquely and centered on the lumbosacral junction. The c-arm is then angled in a cephalad direction, and the L5/S1 disc is brought into view with 25 to 35 degrees of angulation.

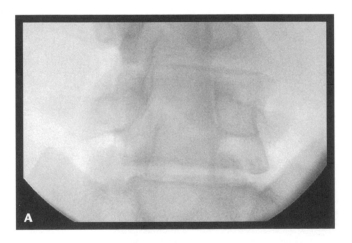
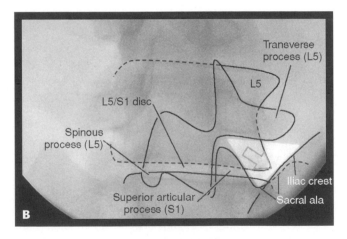

Figure 13-4.
Oblique radiograph of the lumbosacral junction illustrating the triangular window through which the needle passes for superior hypogastric plexus block. **A:** There is a small triangular window through which the needle must pass to reach the anterolateral margin of the lumbosacral junction. **B:** Labeled image. The triangle is bounded superiorly by the transverse process of L5, laterally by the iliac crest, and medially by the L5/S1 facet joint—structures that are readily identified using fluoroscopy. The arrow indicates the target for needle placement for superior hypogastric plexus block.

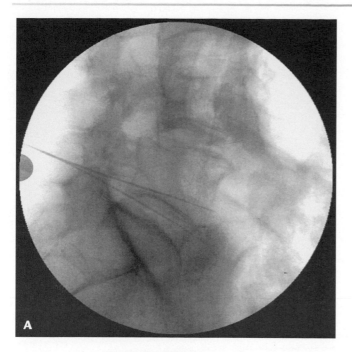
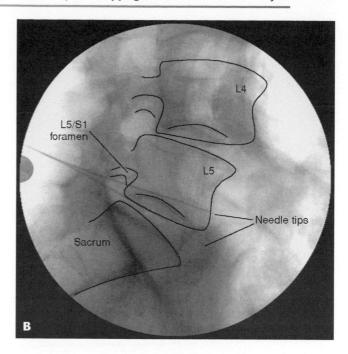

Figure 13-5.
Lateral radiograph of the lumbosacral spine during superior hypogastric plexus block.
A: Two needles are in position over the anterolateral surface of the lumbosacral junction.
The needle tips are aligned with the anterior vertebral margin in the lateral projection.
B: Labeled image. Note the slight cephalad angulation of the x-ray axis causes the needles
to appear one above the other, whereas in the anterior-posterior projection (see Fig. 13-6)
they are at similar levels.

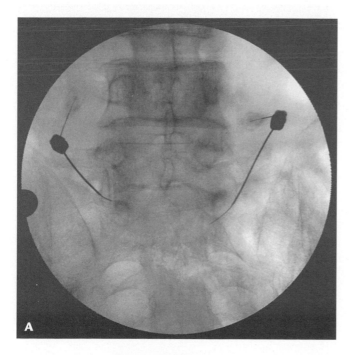
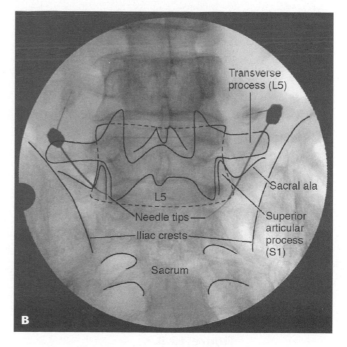

Figure 13-6.
Anterior-Posterior radiograph of the lumbosacral spine during superior hypogastric plexus
block. **A:** Two needles pass obliquely over the sacral ala, where they join with the superior
articular processes of S1. The needle tips are in position over the anterolateral surface of the
L5/S1 intervertebral disc. **B:** Labeled image.

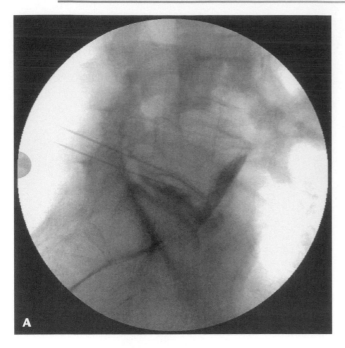
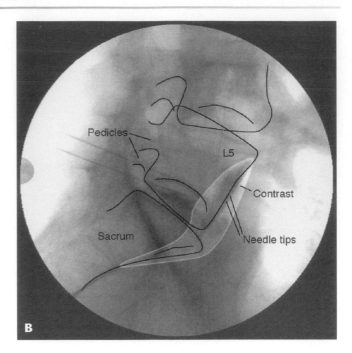

Figure 13-7.
Lateral radiograph of the lumbosacral spine during superior hypogastric plexus block following contrast injection. **A:** Two needles are in position over the anterolateral surface of the lumbosacral junction. The needle tips are aligned with the anterior vertebral margin in the lateral projection. **B:** Labeled image. Note the slight cephalad angulation of the x-ray axis allows the pedicles on each side of midline to be visible. Contrast spreads in a linear fashion over the anterior surface of the L5 vertebral body and the superior portion of the sacrum (*shaded area*).

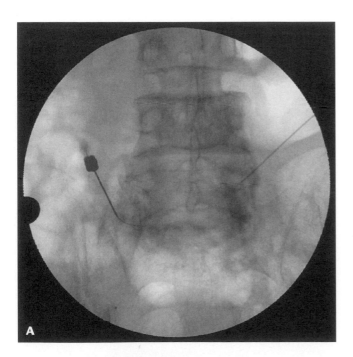
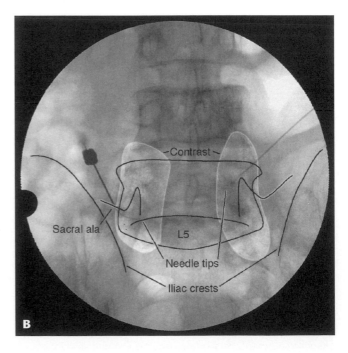

Figure 13-8.
Anterior-Posterior radiograph of the lumbosacral spine during superior hypogastric plexus block following contrast injection. **A:** Two needles pass obliquely over the sacral ala, where they join with the superior articular processes of S1. The needle tips are in position over the anterolateral surface of the L5/S1 intervertebral disc. **B:** Labeled image. Contrast extends along the anterolateral surface of the L5 vertebral body and the superior portion of the sacrum (*shaded areas*).

Superior Hypogastric Neurolysis

In those patients who are candidates for neurolysis who report 50% or more pain reduction with local anesthetic block, neurolysis can be carried out using a technique identical to that used for local anesthetic block, but injecting 5 to 8 mL of 10% phenol on each side. Similar to neurolytic celiac plexus block, the phenol can be dissolved in radiographic contrast (iohexol 180 mg per mL or the equivalent), and the spread can then be monitored during injection to ensure intravascular injection and spread toward the intervertebral foramina are avoided.

Complications

There are only a limited number of reports detailing use of superior hypogastric plexus block, and none have reported complications with this procedure. Due to the close proximity of the iliac vessels, intravascular injection can easily occur.

Acknowledgment: The radiographs used in Figures 13-5–13-8 were generously provided by Paul Kreis, MD, Medical Director and Associate Professor, Division of Pain Medicine, University of California, Davis, Sacramento, CA.

SUGGESTED READINGS

Brown DL. *Atlas of Regional Anesthesia.* 2nd ed. Philadelphia: WB Saunders; 1999:294–302.

Lamer TJ. Sympathetic nerve blocks. In: Brown DL, ed. *Regional Anesthesia and Analgesia.* Philadelphia: WB Saunders; 1996:357–384.

Plancarte R, Amescua C, Patt RB et al. Superior hypogastric plexus block for pelvic cancer pain. *Anesthesiology.* 1990;73:236–239.

Plancarte R, de Leon-Casasola OA, El-Helaly M et al. Neurolytic superior hypogastric plexus block for chronic pelvic pain associated with cancer. *Reg Anesth.* 1997;22:562–568.

Rathmell JP. Sympathetic blocks. In: Rathmell JP, Neal JM, Viscomi CV, eds. *Requisites in Anesthesiology: Regional Anesthesia.* Philadelphia: Elsevier Health Sciences; 2004:128–141.

Intercostal Nerve Block and Neurolysis

Overview

The intercostal nerves supply sensation to the thorax and abdomen. Prior to the widespread adoption of the thoracic epidural approach to provide analgesia following major thoracic and abdominal surgery, multiple intercostal nerve blocks were frequently used to provide postoperative pain control for common abdominal operations such as open cholecystectomy. In the postoperative setting, intercostal nerve block is rarely conducted with radiographic guidance. This is a simple technique that can be performed safely and effectively at the bedside using surface landmarks to guide placement. In contrast, neurolysis of the intercostal nerves has been used to provide long-lasting pain relief for patients with painful metastases involving the chest wall. Use of image-guided injection for neurolysis of the intercostal nerves can ensure that the neurolytic solution is injected at the level of the metastases and in close proximity to the intercostal nerves.

Anatomy

The intercostal nerves arise from the anterior primary rami of the first through twelfth thoracic nerve roots. The thoracic nerve roots exit the intervertebral foramina to enter the paravertebral space (Fig. 14-1). The paravertebral space is bound by the pleura anteromedially, the vertebral body medially, and the transverse spinous processes and paravertebral musculature posteriorly. The ribs traverse this space and form two articulations with the vertebral bodies: the costotransverse articulation, where the rib contacts the transverse process, and the costovertebral articulation, where the head of the rib meets the vertebral body. The thoracic spinal nerve root exits the intervertebral foramen and ramifies into anterior and posterior branches; the anterior branch forms the intercostal nerve. The intercostal nerve traverses laterally to lie in the subcostal groove, a shallow notch along the inferior margin of each rib. Within this groove, the intercostal vein and artery lie in close proximity, just superior to the nerve (Fig. 14-2). This accounts for the high plasma levels of local anesthetic produced with intercostal nerve blocks. The costal groove becomes shallow and disappears altogether some 5 to 8 cm lateral to the posterior midline. The intercostal nerve may lie immediately below the rib margin or closer to the midpoint between ribs as it traverses laterally. The lateral branch of the intercostal nerve rises over the posterolateral chest wall anterior to the posterior axillary line (an imaginary line extending directly inferior from the posterior axillary fold). This is an important factor to understand because intercostal nerve blocks performed anterior to the posterior axillary line may not anesthetize this branch and may produce incomplete truncal anesthesia. The nerves continue anteriorly around the chest wall, ending in the anterior branches. These terminal branches supply sensation to the anterior chest wall.

Patient Selection

Multiple intercostal nerve blocks were frequently used to provide postoperative pain control for common abdominal operations such as open cholecystectomy, but thoracic epidural infusion is simpler and provides effective continuous analgesia. The use of intercostal blocks has also been described for repair of small umbilical hernias, extracorporeal shock wave lithotripsy, and pacemaker insertion. Use of one- or two-level blocks remains an excellent means of providing anesthesia for chest tube insertion. Intercostal nerve block is a simple and effective means for relieving the pain of rib fractures, albeit limited to the duration of local anesthetic effect. Intercostal nerve blocks for treating pain in acute settings are usually carried out without radiographic guidance, using surface landmarks to guide block placement. Intercostal neurolytic blocks using phenol or alcohol have proven effective for treating painful, isolated metastatic lesions involving the ribs, and use of radiographic guidance facilitates safe and effective intercostal neurolysis.

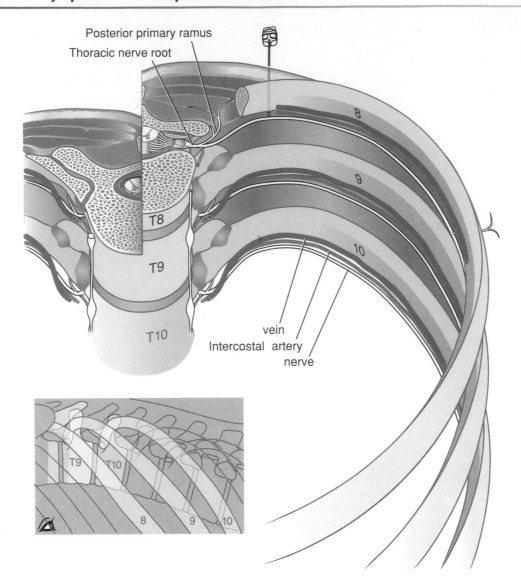

Figure 14-1.

Anatomy of the intercostal nerves. The thoracic nerve roots exit the spinal canal through the intervertebral foramina and divide into anterior and posterior primary rami. The anterior rami course laterally to enter a groove beneath the inferior margin of each rib, where they traverse laterally inferior to the intercostal vein and artery. The posterior cutaneous branch rises in a variable location along the course of the intercostal nerve but always anterior to the posterior axillary line (a line that extends directly inferior from the posterior fold of the axilla). Thus, intercostal nerve block should be carried out medial to the posterior axillary line to ensure the entire sensory distribution of the nerve is blocked. The inset shows the orientation of the diagram.

Positioning

The patient lies prone, with the head turned to one side (Fig. 14-3). The c-arm is centered over the hemithorax on the side to be treated with 15 to 20 degrees of caudal angulation. The intercostal nerves course in a groove beneath the rib, and the caudal angulation ensures the needle will traverse cephalad beneath the rib margin toward the nerve.

Block Technique

The intercostal nerves can be blocked anywhere along their course from the paravertebral region to the anterior chest wall. To obtain complete anesthesia along the trunk within the distribution of a given intercostal nerve, the nerve must be blocked before the posterior cutaneous branch arises (posterior to the posterior axillary line, see Fig. 14-1). Access to the intercostal nerves is blocked by the overlying

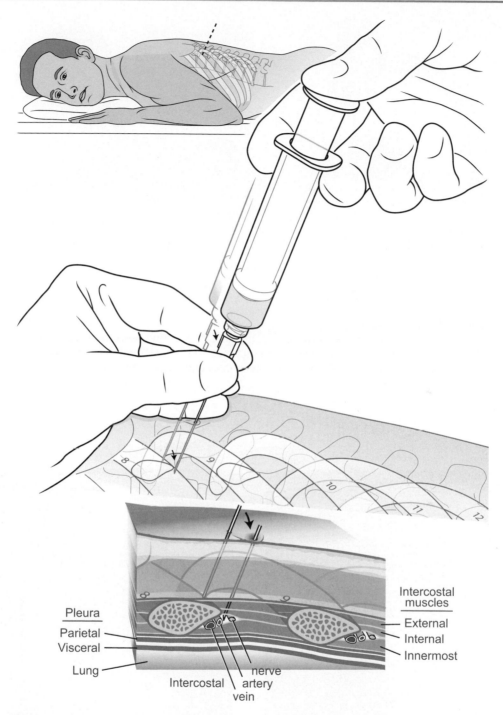

Figure 14-2.
Technique for intercostal nerve block. The needle is advanced with 15 to 20 degrees of cephalad angulation and is first seated on the inferior margin of the rib. The needle is then walked off the inferior rib margin while maintaining the same cephalad angulation of the needle and advanced 2 to 3 mm to lie adjacent to the intercostal nerve. The intercostal nerve lies inferior to the intercostal vein and artery, between the internal and innermost intercostal muscles.

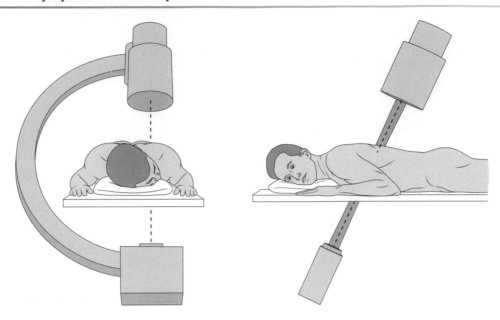

Figure 14-3.
Patient position for intercostal nerve block. The patient lies prone, with the head turned to one side. The c-arm is centered over the hemithorax to be treated with 15 to 20 degrees of caudal angulation to ensure the needle passes in a caudal-to-cephalad direction beneath the inferior margin of the rib.

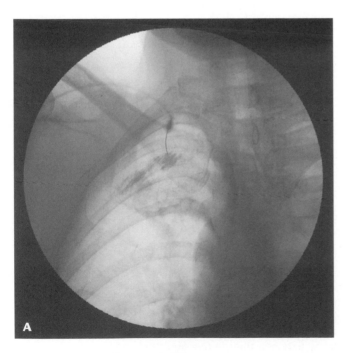

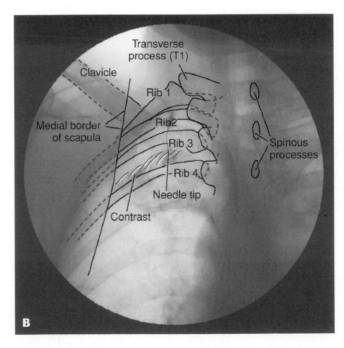

Figure 14-4.
Anterior-Posterior radiograph of the chest during intercostal nerve block demonstrating intramuscular injection. **A:** A needle is in position just inferior to the inferior margin of the third rib, approximately 5 cm from midline. One milliliter of radiographic contrast has been injected (iohexol 180 mg per mL), and spans the space between the third and fourth ribs with a striated pattern that indicates superficial placement between the external and internal intercostal muscles. The needle should be advanced 2 to 3 mm, and the injection repeated. **B:** Labeled image.

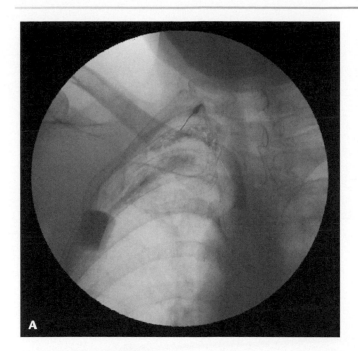
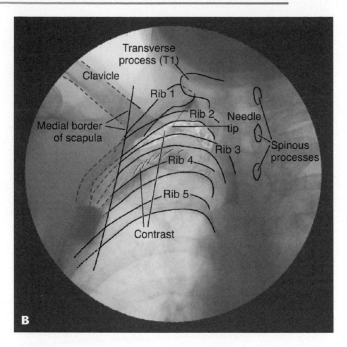

Figure 14-5.
Anterior-Posterior radiograph of the chest during second intercostal neurolysis. **A:** A needle is in position just inferior to the inferior margin of the second rib, approximately 5 cm from midline. Three milliliters of radiographic contrast containing phenol have been injected (10% phenol in iohexol 180 mg per mL). The neurolytic solution has spread along the course of the intercostal nerve, extending medially to the paravertebral space and several centimeters lateral from the point of injection. **B:** Labeled image. Note the residual intramuscular contrast from the first injection (see Fig. 14-4).

scapula above the level of T6 over the posterior chest wall; thus, the block must be carried out medial to the medial scapular border at these levels. Although intercostal blocks can be performed with the patient in nearly any position, the simplest way to perform multiple intercostal blocks is with the patient fully prone. The shoulder can be easily abducted, placing the forearm over the head to swing the scapula laterally and gain access to the upper ribs. The flat portion of each rib is easily palpated several centimeters from midline, and the inferior margin of each rib is marked. The levels to be blocked should be chosen based on the pattern of pain and the location of any chest wall metastases. In the presence of large metastatic lesions, block of the intercostal nerves one level above and below the affected rib may be necessary for effective pain relief.

The block is then carried out sequentially at each level. The inferior margin of each rib to be blocked is identified on fluoroscopy, and a skin wheal of local anesthetic is placed to provide anesthesia of the skin and subcutaneous tissues. A 22-gauge, 1.5-inch needle is inserted just beneath the skin in a plane coaxial with the x-ray path. The rib lies just 1 to 2 cm beneath the skin in the patient of average build, so care must be taken not to advance the needle too far before confirming its trajectory using fluoroscopy. The direction of the needle is

then adjusted to direct the tip toward the inferior margin of the rib and advanced to contact the rib margin. Use of small-gauge needles is advocated by some experts, but because they bend easily, detecting contact with bone is more difficult. Once the needle is in contact with the inferior margin of the rib, the slight cephalad angle of the needle is maintained, and the needle is walked off the inferior margin of the rib, and advanced 2 to 3 mm further (see Fig. 14-2). A small volume of radiographic contrast is then injected to ensure that the needle is in good position and there is no intravascular injection. If the needle is too superficial, the contrast will layer between muscle layers and appear striated (Fig. 14-4). When the needle is adjacent to the intercostal nerve, the contrast typically extends along the inferior margin of the rib, outlining the neurovascular bundle (Fig. 14-5). For temporary or diagnostic intercostal nerve block, 2 to 4 mL of local anesthetic is placed at each level (0.25% or 0.5% bupivacaine). With injection of local anesthetic, the contrast is diluted and spreads along the course of the intercostal nerve (Fig. 14-6). The same procedure is carried out for adjacent levels. The small distance between the rib's inferior margin and the pleura must be emphasized; advancing the needle more than a few millimeters beyond the bony margin may result in pneumothorax (see Fig. 14-2).

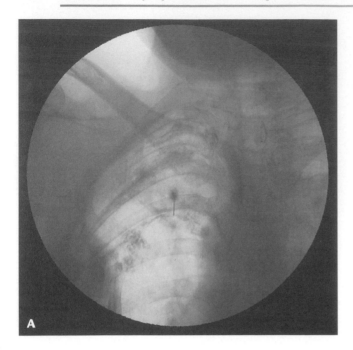
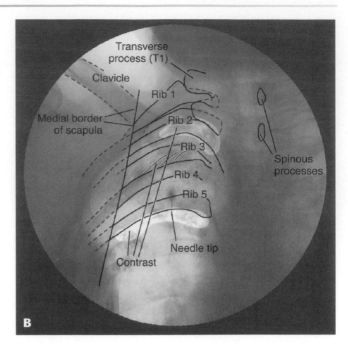

Figure 14-6.

Anterior-Posterior radiograph of the chest during fifth intercostal neurolysis. **A:** A needle is in position just inferior to the inferior margin of the fourth rib, approximately 5 cm from midline. Three milliliters of radiographic contrast containing phenol have been injected (10% phenol in iohexol 180 mg per mL). The neurolytic solution has spread along the course of the intercostal nerve, extending several centimeters medial and lateral from the point of injection. **B:** Labeled image. Note the residual contrast from the first two injections (see Figs. 14-4 and 14-5).

Intercostal Neurolysis

Neurolysis of the intercostal nerves is carried out in the same manner described for intercostal nerve blocks using local anesthetic. Once the needle position has been confirmed with the injection of a small amount of radiographic contrast, the neurolytic solution is placed. Use of 10% phenol in radiographic contrast (e.g., iohexol 180 mg per mL) allows the spread of the injectate to be monitored (see Figs. 14-5 and 14-6). Injection of 2 to 4 mL of neurolytic solution is usually sufficient to produce spread along a 5- to 8-cm segment of the nerve. When intercostal neurolysis is carried out close to the proximal portion of the rib, the contrast will often extend to the paravertebral space and extend through the intervertebral foramen to the lateral epidural space. Epidural neurolysis is well described. In fact, extension of the contrast into the epidural space is unlikely to cause adverse effects and may well improve the results of neurolysis.

Complications

Because of the close proximity of vascular structures to the intercostal nerves, there is a significant risk of direct intravascular injection and vascular uptake during each block. Intercostal nerve blocks result in plasma concentrations of local anesthetic greater than any other peripheral nerve block, and care must be taken not to exceed total doses that may lead to systemic toxicity (see Table 4-3). Thus, close attention must be paid to the total local anesthetic dose delivered and to adequate monitoring, intravenous access, and ready availability of resuscitation equipment and drugs.

Pneumothorax can occur, but the incidence is low. Centers with extensive experience using intercostal nerve blocks for postoperative analgesia have reported significant pneumothorax in less than 0.1% of cases. The incidence is clinically insignificant, but radiographically demonstrable pneumothorax is somewhat higher (0.42%). Treatment of most pneumothoraces should be conservative, with observation and administration of oxygen, which will also aid reabsorption. Needle aspiration or chest tube drainage is rarely necessary and should be reserved only for patients with symptomatic pneumothorax.

Worsening of pain can arise during intercostal neurolysis and is likely the result of incomplete neurolysis of the treated intercostal nerve. Such patients typically report worsened pain in the distribution of the treated intercostal nerve, and may develop signs and symptoms of neuropathic pain, including burning or lancinating pain and allodynia in the affected region. Although this exacerbation of pain following intercostal neurolysis is usually self-limited, repeat neurolysis may be necessary to reduce or eliminate the pain, and pain may persist even after repeat neurolysis. There is at least one case report of spinal cord injury following intercostal neurolysis, but the mechanism of injury is not clear.

SUGGESTED READINGS

Brown DL. *Atlas of Regional Anesthesia*. 2nd ed. Philadelphia: WB Saunders; 1999:240–246.

Kopacz DJ. Regional anesthesia of the trunk. In: Brown DL, ed. *Regional Anesthesia and Analgesia*. Philadelphia: WB Saunders; 1996:292–318.

Kowalewski R, Schurch B, Hodler J et al. Persistent paraplegia after an aqueous 7.5% phenol solution to the anterior motor root for intercostal neurolysis: a case report. *Arch Phys Med Rehabil*. 2002;83: 283–285.

Neumann M, Raj PP. Thoracoabdominal pain. In: Raj PP, ed. *Practical Management of Pain*. 3rd ed. St. Louis, MO: Mosby; 2000:618–629.

IMPLANTABLE DEVICES

CHAPTER 15

Implantable Spinal Drug Delivery System Placement

Overview

Intrathecal morphine and other opioids are now widely used as useful adjuncts in the treatment of acute and chronic pain, and a number of agents show promise as analgesic agents with spinal selectivity. Continuous delivery of analgesic agents at the spinal level can be carried out using percutaneous epidural or intrathecal catheters, but vulnerability to infection and the cost of external systems typically limits them to short-term use (<6 weeks). Reliable implanted drug delivery systems are now available that make long-term delivery of medications to the intrathecal space feasible. These systems are comprised of a drug reservoir/pump implanted within the subcutaneous tissue of the abdominal wall, which is refilled periodically through an access port. The pump may be a fixed-rate, constant flow device or a variable-rate pump that can be programmed using a wireless radiofrequency transmitter similar to those used for implanted cardiac pacemakers.

Anatomy

The intrathecal catheter is placed directly within the cerebrospinal fluid (CSF) of the lumbar cistern by advancing a needle between vertebral laminae at the L2/L3 level or below. Direct delivery of the opioid at the spinal level corresponding to the dermatome(s) in which the patient is experiencing pain may improve analgesia, particularly when local anesthetics or lipophilic opioids (e.g., fentanyl or sufentanil) are used. Thus, some practitioners have advocated threading the catheter cephalad to the appropriate dermatome. In more recent years, reports of inflammatory mass formation surrounding the catheter tip of some chronic indwelling intrathecal catheters have appeared. These inflammatory masses often presented with gradual neurologic deterioration caused by spinal cord compression. Many physicians now recommend that implanted intrathecal catheters be placed only within the lumbar cistern below the conus medullaris (below ~L2), where the appearance of an inflammatory mass is less likely to directly impinge on the spinal cord.

Patient Selection

Patient selection for intraspinal pain therapy is empiric and remains the subject of debate. In general, intrathecal drug delivery is reserved for patients with severe pain that does not respond to conservative treatment. In patients with cancer-related pain, most will have ongoing pain despite appropriate oral opioid therapy, or they may have developed intolerable side effects related to these medications. Randomized controlled trials comparing maximal medical therapy with intrathecal drug delivery for cancer-related pain have demonstrated improved pain control and reduction in opioid-related side effects in those who received intrathecal pain therapy. Intrathecal drug delivery has also been widely used for noncancer pain, particularly for the treatment of chronic low back pain. Use of this therapy in noncancer pain has not been subject to controlled trials.

Once a patient is selected for intrathecal therapy, a trial is carried out. Most physicians now conduct trials by placing a temporary, percutaneous intrathecal catheter and infusing the analgesic agent over several days to judge the effectiveness of this therapy *before* a permanent system is implanted. Some carry out the trial of intrathecal therapy using a single dose or by using a continuous epidural infusion. The most common analgesic agent used for spinal delivery is morphine; this remains the only opioid approved by the U.S. Food and Drug Administration for intrathecal use.

Positioning

Before the procedure, discuss with the patient the location of the pocket for the intrathecal pump. Most devices are large, and the only region suitable for placement is the left

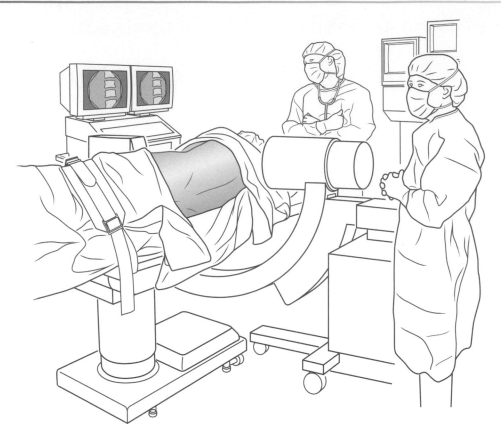

Figure 15-1.
View of typical operating room arrangement during intrathecal implantation. The patient is placed in the lateral position with the c-arm in place for a cross-table anterior-posterior view of the lumbar spine.

or right lower quadrants of the abdomen. Once the site is determined, mark the proposed skin incision with a permanent marker while the patient is in the sitting position. The position of the pocket on the abdominal wall is deceptively difficult to determine once the patient is lying on his or her side. If the location is not marked, the pocket is often placed too far lateral within the abdominal wall.

Implantation of an intrathecal drug delivery system is a minor surgical procedure that is carried out in the operating room using aseptic precautions, including skin preparation, sterile draping, and use of full surgical attire (Fig. 15-1). The procedure can be conducted under either local anesthesia or general anesthesia using dedicated anesthesia personnel. Performing the initial spinal catheter placement under general anesthesia is controversial, and concerns about neural injury are similar to performing any neuraxial technique under general anesthesia.

The patient is positioned on a radiolucent table in the lateral decubitus position with the patient's side for the pump pocket nondependent (see Fig. 15-1). The arms are extended at the shoulders and secured in position so they are well away from the surgical field. The skin is prepared, and sterile drapes are applied. The radiographic c-arm is then positioned across the lumbar region to provide a cross-

table anterior-posterior (AP) view of the lumbar spine. Care must be taken to ensure that the x-ray view is not rotated by observing that the spinous processes are in the midline, halfway between the vertebral pedicles (Fig. 15-2).

Surgical Technique

The L3/L4, L4/L5, or L5/S1 interspace is identified using fluoroscopy. The spinal needle supplied by the intrathecal device manufacturer must be used to ensure that the catheter will advance through the needle without damage. The needle is advanced using a paramedian approach starting 1 to 1.5 cm lateral to the spinous processes and just inferior to the superior margin of the lamina that forms the inferior border of the interspace you plan to enter (see Fig. 15-2). The needle is directed to enter the spinal space in the midline; after dural penetration, the stylette is removed to ensure adequate flow of CSF (Fig. 15-3). Using fluoroscopic guidance, the spinal catheter is advanced through the needle until the tip is well into the spinal space but below L2 within the lumbar cistern (Fig. 15-4). Position of the catheter tip is verified using fluoroscopy in the AP and lateral planes (Figs. 15-5 and 15-6). The needle is then withdrawn slightly (~1 to 2 cm) but left in

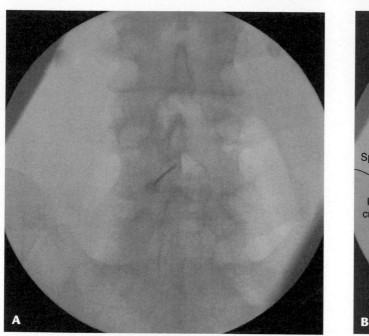
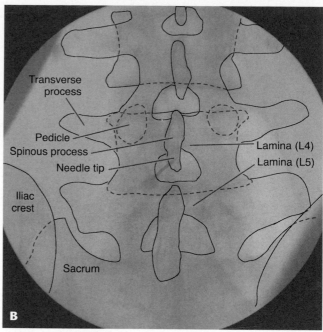

Figure 15-2.
A: Initial spinal needle placement via the L4/L5 interspace using a left paramedian approach. **B:** Labeled image.

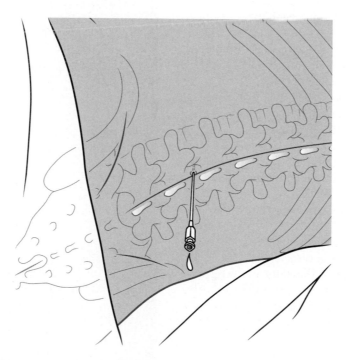

Figure 15-3.
Free flow of cerebrospinal fluid indicates intrathecal location.

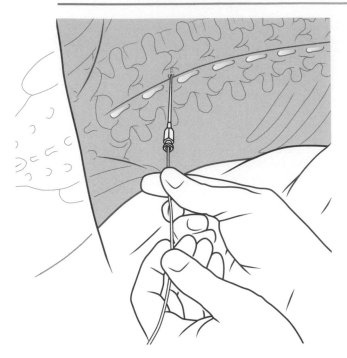

Figure 15-4.
Intrathecal catheter placement through the spinal needle under fluoroscopic guidance.

If the pocket is placed cephalad to the incision, the weight of the device on the suture line is likely to cause wound dehiscence. In many patients, the blunt dissection can be accomplished using gentle but firm pressure with the fingers. It is simpler and less traumatic to use a small pair of surgical scissors to perform the blunt dissection using repeated opening (*not closing or cutting*) motions. After creating the pocket, the pump is placed in the pocket to ensure the pocket is large enough. The pump should fit completely within the pocket without any part of the device extending beneath the incision. With the device in place, the wound margins must fall into close apposition. There should be no tension on the sutures during closure of the incision or the wound is likely to dehisce.

After pocket creation is completed, a tunneling device is extended within the subcutaneous tissues between the paraspinous incision and the pocket (Fig. 15-13). The catheter is then advanced through the tunnel (most tunneling devices place a hollow plastic sleeve in the subcutaneous tissue through which the catheter can be advanced from the

place around the catheter within the subcutaneous tissues to protect the catheter during the subsequent dissection (Fig. 15-7). The catheter is secured to the surgical field using a small clamp to ensure it does not fall outside the sterile field (see Fig. 15-7).

A 5- to 8-cm incision parallel to the axis of the spine is extended from just cephalad to just caudad to the needle, extending directly through the needle's skin entry point (Fig. 15-8). The subcutaneous tissues are divided using blunt dissection until the lumbar paraspinous fascia is visible surrounding the needle shaft. A purse-string suture is created within the fascia surrounding the needle shaft (Fig. 15-9). This suture is used to tighten the fascia around the catheter and prevent backflow of CSF that may lead to a chronic subcutaneous CSF collection. The needle and stylette are removed simultaneously, using care not to dislodge the spinal catheter (Fig. 15-10). Free flow of CSF from the catheter should be evident after the stylette is removed; if there is no CSF flowing from the catheter, a blunt needle can be inserted within the end of the catheter and gentle aspiration used to ensure the catheter remains within the thecal sac. If CSF cannot be aspirated from the catheter, it should be removed and replaced. The catheter is then secured to the paraspinous fascia using a specific anchoring device supplied by the manufacturer (Fig. 15-11).

Attention is now turned to creating the pocket within the patient's abdominal wall. A 10- to 12-cm transverse incision is made along the previously marked line, and a subcutaneous pocket is created using blunt dissection (Fig. 15-12). The pocket should always be created caudad to the incision.

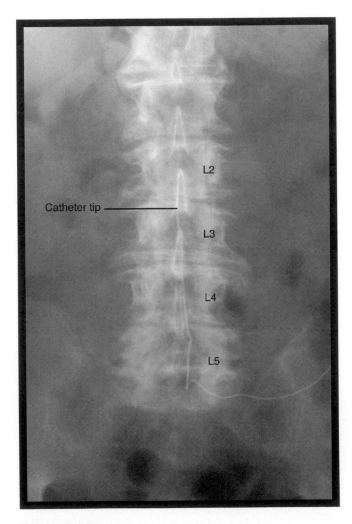

Figure 15-5.
Anterior-Posterior radiograph of the intrathecal catheter tip (*arrow*) in final position with tip adjacent to the L2/L3 intervertebral disc.

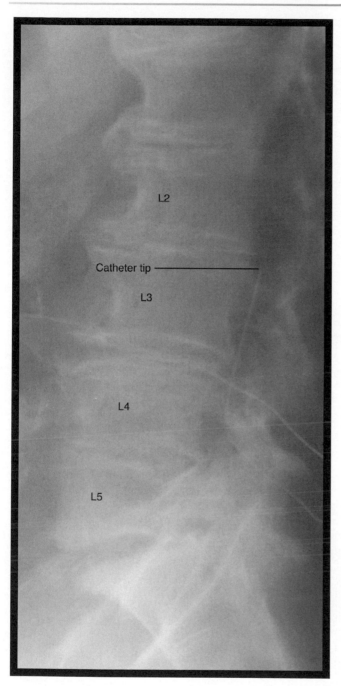

Figure 15-6.
Lateral radiograph of the intrathecal catheter tip (*arrow*) in final position with tip adjacent to the L2/L3 intervertebral disc.

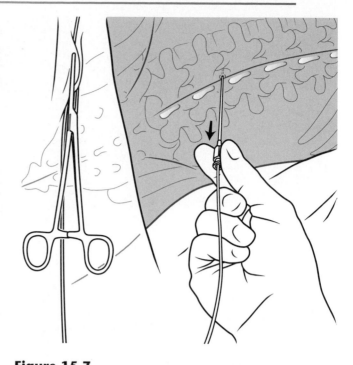

Figure 15-7.
After confirming the final position of the catheter tip, the spinal needle is withdrawn about 1 cm to lie in the subcutaneous tissue, and the proximal portion of the catheter is fastened to the surgical field. Leaving the needle in place protects the catheter during subsequent dissection.

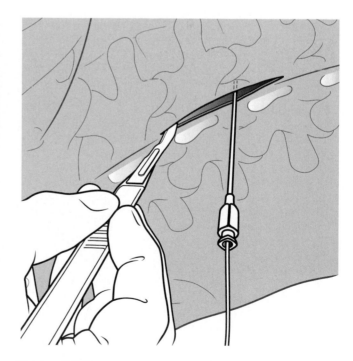

Figure 15-8.
A cephalad-caudad incision is made through the skin and subcutaneous tissues; the incision extends above and below the needle entry point. Using blunt dissection, the skin and subcutaneous tissues are further divided until the lumbar paravertebral fascia is exposed.

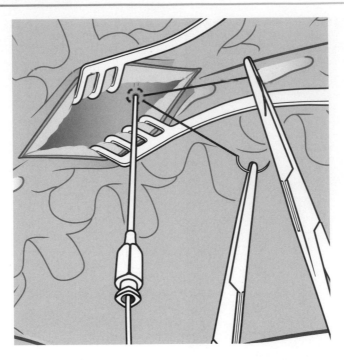

Figure 15-9.
A purse-string suture is placed around the base of the needle within the paravertebral fascia. This suture reduces the likelihood that cerebrospinal fluid (CSF) will track back along the catheter and result in a subcutaneous CSF collection.

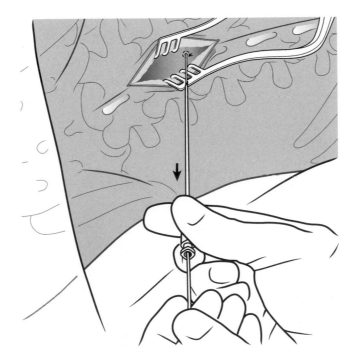

Figure 15-10.
The needle and stylette are removed together while holding the catheter firmly in position.

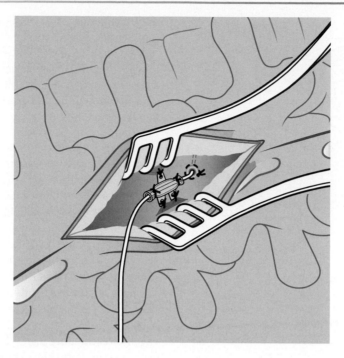

Figure 15-11.
The catheter is secured to the paravertebral fascia using an anchoring device supplied by the manufacturer.

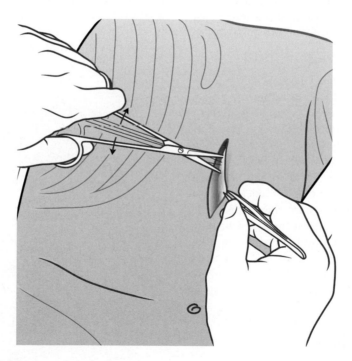

Figure 15-12.
A transverse incision is created in the abdominal wall midway between the umbilicus and the anterior axillary line and a pocket of sufficient size is made to accommodate the pump using blunt dissection. The blunt dissection can be accomplished using the fingertips or by using surgical scissors and a repeated spreading (rather than cutting) motion.

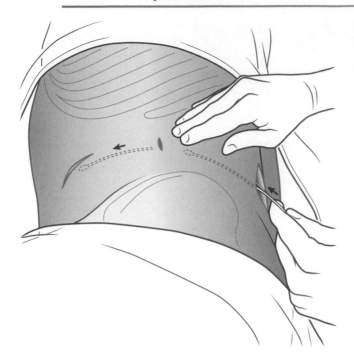

Figure 15-13.
A tunneling device provided by the manufacturer is used to position the catheter within the subcutaneous tissue between the paravertebral incision and the abdominal pump pocket. In large patients, the tunneling often requires two segments; the first segment between the paravertebral incision and a small transverse incision in the mid-axillary line, and a second segment from the mid-axillary line to the abdominal pump pocket.

patient's back to pump pocket). The catheter is then trimmed to a length that allows for a small loop of catheter to remain deep to the pump and attach to the pump. The pump is placed in the pocket with a loop of catheter deep to the device (Fig. 15-14). This loop allows for patient movement without placing tension on the distal catheter and causing it to be pulled from the thecal sac. Two or more sutures should be placed through the suture loops or mesh enclosure surrounding the pump and used to secure the pump to the abdominal fascia. These simple retaining sutures prevent the pump from rotating or flipping within the pocket. The skin incisions are then closed in two layers: a series of interrupted subcutaneous sutures to securely close the fascia overlying the pump, and the catheter followed by a skin closure using suture or staples (Fig. 15-15).

Permanent Epidural Catheter Placement

For placement of a permanent epidural catheter, patient positioning and use of fluoroscopy are similar to those described for intrathecal catheter placement. The interspace of entry will vary with the dermatomes that are to be covered, particularly if local anesthetic solution is to be used. A typical loss-of-resistance technique is used to identify the epidural space, and a silastic catheter is threaded into the epidural space. A paraspinous incision is created, and the catheter is secured to

the paraspinous fascia as described previously for intrathecal catheter placement.

Two types of permanent epidural systems are available: a totally implanted system using a subcutaneous port that is accessed using a needle placed into the port through the skin, and a percutaneous catheter that is tunneled subcutaneously but exits the skin to be connected directly to an external infusion device.

To place a permanent epidural with a subcutaneous port, a 6- to 8-cm transverse incision is made overlying the costal margin halfway between the xiphoid process and the anterior axillary line. A pocket is created overlying the rib cage using blunt dissection (Fig. 15-16). The catheter is then tunneled from the paraspinous region to the pocket as described previously for intrathecal catheter placement and secured to the port. The port must then be sutured securely to the fascia over the rib cage. Care must be taken to ensure the port is secured firmly in a region that overlies the rib cage; if the port migrates inferiorly to lie over the abdomen, it becomes difficult to access. The rigid support of the rib cage holds the port firmly from behind, allowing for easier access to the port. The skin incisions are then closed in two layers: a series of interrupted subcutaneous sutures to securely close the fascia overlying the catheter, followed by a skin closure using suture or staples.

To place a permanent epidural without a subcutaneous port, a tunneling device is extended from the paraspinous incision to the right upper abdominal quadrant, just inferior to the costal margin. A small incision (~0.5 cm) is made to allow the tunneling device to exit the skin. Percutaneous

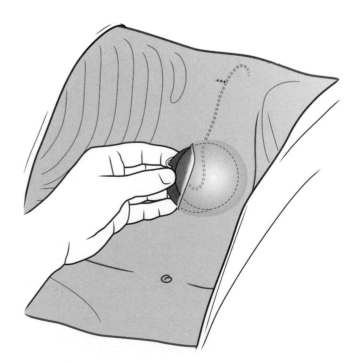

Figure 15-14.
After ensuring good hemostasis, the pump is placed within the pocket.

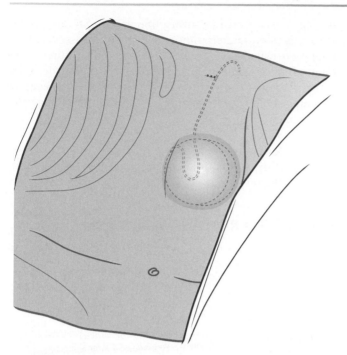

Figure 15-15.
The abdominal and paravertebral incisions are then closed in two layers: a layer of interrupted, absorbable suture within the subcutaneous tissue overlying the pump and catheter, and a separate layer within the skin.

epidural catheters are supplied in two parts: the proximal portion of the catheter that is placed within the epidural space, and the distal portion of the catheter that enters the abdominal wall and connects with the distal portion of the catheter. The distal portion of the catheter is now secured to the tunneling device and pulled through the incision in the abdominal wall subcutaneously to emerge from the paraspinous incision (Fig. 15-17). Many catheters are supplied with an antibiotic-impregnated cuff that is designed to arrest entry of bacteria along the track of the catheter. This cuff should be placed about 1 cm from the catheter's exit site along the subcutaneous catheter track. The proximal and distal portions of the catheter are then trimmed, leaving enough catheter length to ensure there is no traction on the catheter with movement. The two ends of the catheter are connected using a stainless steel union supplied by the manufacturer and sutured securely. The paraspinous skin incision is then closed in two layers: a series of interrupted subcutaneous sutures to securely close the fascia overlying the catheter, followed by a skin closure using suture or staples. The skin incision at the epidural catheter's exit site in the right upper quadrant is closed around the base of the catheter using one or two simple, interrupted sutures.

Complications

Bleeding and infection are risks inherent to all open surgical procedures. Bleeding within the pump pocket can lead

to a hematoma surrounding the pump that may require surgical drainage. Bleeding along the subcutaneous tunneling track often causes significant bruising in the region but rarely requires treatment. Similar to other neuraxial techniques, bleeding within the epidural space can lead to significant neural compression. Signs of infection within the pump pocket typically occur within 10 to 14 days following implantation but may occur at any time. Some practitioners have reported successful treatment of superficial infections of the area overlying the pocket with oral antibiotics aimed at the offending organism and close observation alone. However, infections within the pocket or along the catheter's subcutaneous course almost universally require removal of all implanted hardware and treatment with parenteral antibiotics to eradicate infection. Catheter and deep tissue infections can extend to involve the neuraxis, resulting in epidural abscess formation and/or meningitis. Permanent epidural catheters without subcutaneous ports have a higher infection rate than those with ports in the first weeks after placement, but both systems have a similar, high rate of infection when left in place for more than 6 to 8 weeks.

Spinal cord injury during initial catheter placement has been reported. Most practitioners recommend placing the catheter only in the awake patient so the patient can report

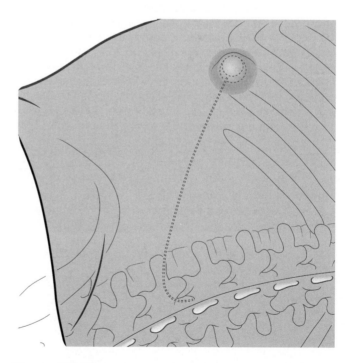

Figure 15-16.
Placement of a permanent epidural catheter with a subcutaneous access port. The epidural catheter is placed and tunneled to a pocket over the costal margin. The port is connected to the epidural catheter and sutured to the fascia overlying the inferior rib cage. The port must lie firmly in place over the ribs rather than the abdominal wall; without the support of the firm rib cage behind the port, it will be difficult to access.

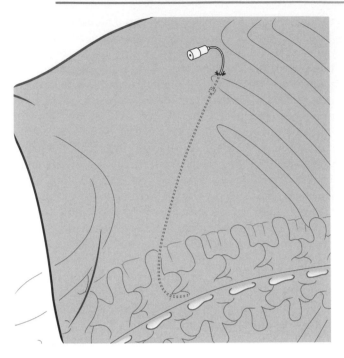

Figure 15-17.
Placement of a permanent percutaneous, tunneled epidural catheter. This type of catheter is typically supplied in two pieces: a distal, epidural portion, and a proximal catheter length with a subcutaneous antibiotic-impregnated cuff and external access port. After placement of the epidural catheter and dissection through a paravertebral incision, the proximal catheter is tunneled from the costal margin to the paravertebral incision, and the catheter is pulled into the subcutaneous tissues until the antibiotic-impregnated cuff lies 1 to 2 cm from the chest wall incision within the subcutaneous tissue. The catheter segments are then trimmed, joined together using a connector supplied by the manufacturer, and secured to the paravertebral fascia. The skin entry site on the chest wall is secured around the exiting catheter using interrupted sutures.

paresthesiae during needle placement. The catheter can be placed incorrectly within the subdural compartment or the intrathecal epidural space.

Wound dehiscence and migration are infrequent problems. Ensuring the size of the pocket is sufficient to

prevent tension on the suture line at the time of wound closure is essential to minimize the risk of dehiscence. Port migration usually occurs because retaining sutures were omitted at the time of placement. Placing two or more sutures through the suture loops on the port and securely fastening them to the abdominal fascia will minimize the risk of migration.

Subcutaneous collection of fluid surrounding the port (seroma formation) can be problematic. Percutaneous drainage of the sterile fluid collection is often successful in resolving the problem.

SUGGESTED READINGS

Bennett G, Burchiel K, Buchser E et al. Clinical guidelines for intraspinal infusion: report of an expert panel. PolyAnalgesic Consensus Conference 2000. *J Pain Symptom Manage.* 2000;20:S37–S43.

Bennett G, Serafini M, Burchiel K et al. Evidence-based review of the literature on intrathecal delivery of pain medication. *J Pain Symptom Manage.* 2000;20:S12–S36.

Follett KA, Naumann CP. A prospective study of catheter-related complications of intrathecal drug delivery systems. *J Pain Symptom Manage.* 2000;19:209–215.

Hassenbusch SJ, Portenoy RK, Cousins M et al. PolyAnalgesic Consensus Conference 2003: an update on the management of pain by intraspinal drug delivery—report of an expert panel. *J Pain Symptom Manage.* 2004;27:540–563.

Kedlaya D, Reynolds L, Waldman S. Epidural and intrathecal analgesia for cancer pain. *Best Pract Res Clin Anaesthesiol.* 2002;16:651–665.

Kumar K, Hunter G, Demeria DD. Treatment of chronic pain by using intrathecal drug therapy compared with conventional pain therapies: a cost-effectiveness analysis. *J Neurosurg.* 2002;97:803–810.

Prager JP. Neuraxial medication delivery: the development and maturity of a concept for treating chronic pain of spinal origin. *Spine.* 2002;27: 2,593–2,605.

Rainov NG, Heidecke V, Burkert W. Long-term intrathecal infusion of drug combinations for chronic back and leg pain. *J Pain Symptom Manage.* 2001;22:862–871.

Smith TJ, Staats PS, Deer T et al. Randomized clinical trial of an implantable drug delivery system compared with comprehensive medical management for refractory cancer pain: impact on pain, drug-related toxicity, and survival. *J Clin Oncol.* 2002;20:4,040–4,049.

Yaksh TL, Hassenbusch S, Burchiel K et al. Inflammatory masses associated with intrathecal drug infusion: a review of preclinical evidence and human data. *Pain Med.* 2002;3:300–312.

Spinal Cord Stimulation System Placement

Overview

The idea that direct stimulation of the ascending sensory tracts within the spinal cord might interfere with the perception of chronic pain is founded in everyday observations. We are all familiar with the fact that rubbing an area that has just been injured seemingly reduces the amount of pain coming from the injured region. The advent of transcutaneous electrical nerve stimulation (TENS), whereby a light, pleasant electrical current is passed through surface electrodes in the region of ongoing pain, reinforced the observation that stimulation of sensory pathways reduces pain perception in chronic pain states. In 1965, Patrick Wall, a neurophysiologist exploring the basic physiologic mechanisms of pain transmission, and Ronald Melzack, a psychologist working with patients who had chronic pain, together proposed the *gate control theory* to explain how non-noxious stimulation can reduce pain perception. In their theory, they proposed that second-order neurons at the level of the spinal cord dorsal horn act as a "gate" through which noxious stimuli must pass to reach higher centers in the brain and be perceived as pain. If these same neurons receive input from other sensory fibers entering via the same set of neurons within the spinal cord, the non-noxious input can effectively close the gate, preventing simultaneous transmission of noxious input. Thus, the light touch of rubbing an injured region or the pleasant electrical stimulation of TENS closes the gate to the noxious input of chronic pain. From this theory, investigators developed the concept of direct activation of the ascending fibers within the dorsal columns that transmit nonpainful cutaneous stimuli (e.g., light touch) as a means of treating chronic pain. We have learned much about the anatomy and physiology of pain perception since the gate control theory was first proposed. It is unlikely that the simplistic notion of a gate within the dorsal horn is responsible for our observations, but the theory served as a useful concept in the development of spinal cord stimulation (SCS). Both the peripheral nerve fibers and the second-order neurons within the dorsal horn responsible for pain transmission become sensitized following injury, and anatomic changes, cell death, and altered gene expression are all likely to have a role in chronic pain. Direct electrical stimulation of the dorsal columns (referred to as SCS or dorsal column stimulation) has proven effective, particularly in the treatment of chronic radicular pain. The mechanism remains unclear, but direct electrical stimulation within the dorsal columns may produce retrograde changes within the ascending sensory fibers that modulate the intensity of incoming noxious stimuli.

Anatomy

The epidural SCS lead is placed directly within the dorsal epidural space just to one side of midline using a paramedian, interlaminar approach. Entry into the epidural space is performed several levels below the final intended level of lead placement. Typically, leads for stimulation of the low back and lower extremities are placed via the L1/L2 interspace, and those for upper-extremity stimulation are placed via the C7/T1 interspace. Investigators have mapped the patterns of electrical stimulation of the dorsal columns and the corresponding patterns of coverage reported by patients with leads in various locations. In general, the epidural lead must be positioned 2 to 3 mm to the left or right of midline on the same side as the painful region to be covered. For lower-extremity stimulation, successful coverage is usually achieved by placing the lead between the T8 and T10 vertebral levels, whereas upper-extremity stimulation usually requires lead placement between the occiput and C3 vertebral levels. If the lead ventures too far from midline, uncomfortable stimulation of the exiting nerve roots will result. If the lead is placed too low, overlying the conus medullaris (at or below ~L1/L2), unpredictable patterns of stimulation may result. In the region of the conus, the fibers of the dorsal columns do not lie parallel to the midline; rather, they arc from the corresponding nerve root entering the spinal cord toward their eventual paramedian location several levels cephalad.

Patient Selection

Patient selection for SCS is empiric and remains a subject of some debate. In general, SCS is reserved for patients with severe pain that does not respond to conservative treatment. The pain responds best when relatively well localized because success of SCS depends on the ability to cover the entire painful region with electrical stimulation. Attaining adequate coverage is more difficult when pain is bilateral, often requiring two leads, one to each side of midline. When the pain is diffuse, it may be impossible to get effective coverage with stimulation using SCS. Among the best-established indications for SCS is chronic radicular pain with or without radiculopathy in either the upper or the lower extremities. Use of SCS to treat chronic, axial low back pain has been less satisfactory, but more recent results seem to be improving with the advent of dual lead systems and electrode arrays that allow for a broad area of stimulation. Randomized controlled trials comparing SCS with repeat surgery for patients with failed back surgery syndrome have demonstrated greater success in attaining satisfactory pain relief in those treated with SCS. More recent, small randomized controlled trials also suggest significant improvement in pain relief and physical function in patients with CRPS who are treated with SCS in conjunction with physical therapy when compared with physical therapy alone. Prospective observational studies indicate an overall success rate of about 50% (defined as at least 50% pain reduction and ongoing use of SCS 5 years following implantation) in mixed groups of patients with ongoing low back and/or extremity pain following prior lumbar surgery. The usefulness of psychological screening prior to SCS remains controversial; some investigators have suggested that screening for patients with personality disorders, somatoform disorder, or hypochondriasis may improve success rate of SCS.

Once a patient is selected for therapy with SCS, a trial is carried out. Most physicians now conduct trials by placing a temporary, percutaneous epidural lead and conducting the screening using an external device as an outpatient procedure to judge the effectiveness of this therapy before a permanent system is implanted. Some carry out the trial of SCS using a surgically implanted lead that is tunneled using a lead extension that exits percutaneously. The strictly percutaneous trial lead is simpler to place and does not require full operating room setup, but the lead must be removed and replaced surgically following a successful trial. The surgically implanted trial lead requires placement in the operating room, and surgical removal if the trial is unsuccessful. If the trial is successful, the implanted trial lead can remain, and the second procedure to place the impulse generator is brief, not requiring the placement of a new epidural lead. In either case, after successful trial stimulation, a permanent system is placed and the lead is positioned to produce the same pattern of stimulation that afforded pain relief during the period of trial stimulation.

Positioning

Placement of a percutaneous trial spinal cord stimulator lead can be carried out in any location that is suitable for epidural catheter placement. This may be done in the operating room, but it can easily and safely be carried out in any location that allows for adequate sterile preparation of the skin and draping of the operative field and that has fluoroscopy available to guide anatomic placement. Using a strictly percutaneous trial, the trial lead is placed in the same fashion used for permanent lead placement, but the lead is secured to the skin without any incision for the trial period.

Before permanent spinal cord stimulator implantation, discuss with the patient the location of the pocket for the impulse generator. The regions most suitable for placement are the lower quadrant of the abdomen or the lateral aspect of the buttock. Once the site is determined, mark the proposed skin incision with a permanent marker while the patient is in the sitting position. The position of the pocket is deceptively difficult to determine once the patient is lying on his or her side. If the location is not marked, the pocket is often placed too far lateral within the abdominal wall. Placement of the impulse generator within the buttock allows for the entire procedure to be carried out with the patient in the prone position and simplifies the operation by obviating the need to turn from the prone to lateral position halfway through implantation.

Implantation of a spinal cord stimulator lead and impulse generator is a minor surgical procedure that is carried out in the operating room using aseptic precautions, including skin preparation, sterile draping, and use of full surgical attire (Fig. 16-1). The procedure must be conducted using local anesthesia and light enough sedation that the patient can report where they feel the electrical stimulation during lead placement.

The patient is positioned on a radiolucent table in the prone position (see Fig. 16-1). Initial lead placement can be carried out with the patient in a lateral decubitus position; however, even small degrees of rotation along the spinal axis can make positioning of the lead difficult. The arms are extended upward so they are in a position of comfort well away from the surgical field. The skin is prepared, and sterile drapes are applied. For stimulation in the low back and lower extremities, the radiographic c-arm is positioned directly over the thoracolumbar junction to provide an anteroposterior view of the spine. Care must be taken to ensure the x-ray view is not rotated by observing that the spinous processes are in the midline, halfway between the vertebral pedicles (Fig. 16-2).

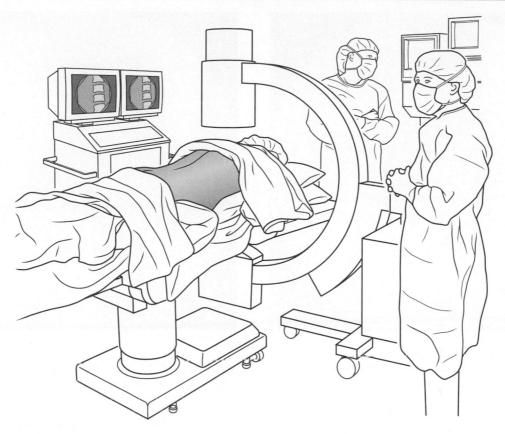

Figure 16-1.
View of typical operating room arrangement during spinal cord stimulator implantation.
The patient is placed in the prone position with the c-arm in place for an anterior-posterior
view of the thoracolumbar spine.

Surgical Technique

The L1/L2 interspace is identified using fluoroscopy. The epidural needle supplied by the device manufacturer must be used to ensure the lead will advance through the needle without damage. The needle is advanced using a paramedian approach, starting 1 to 1.5 cm lateral to the spinous processes and somewhat caudad to the interspace to be entered. The needle is directed to enter the spinal space in the midline, with an angle of entry no greater than 45 degrees from the plane of the epidural space (Figs. 16-2 and 16-3). If the angle of attack of the needle on initial entry into to the epidural space is too great, the epidural lead will be difficult to thread as it negotiates the steep angle between the needle and the plane of the epidural space. The epidural space is identified using a loss-of-resistance (LOR) technique. The electrode is then advanced through the needle and is directed to remain to one side of midline in the dorsal epidural space as it is threaded cephalad under fluoroscopic guidance (Figs. 16-4 and 16-5). The electrode contains a wire stylette with a slight angulation at the tip; gentle rotation of the electrode as it is advanced allows the operator to direct the electrode's path within the epidural space (Fig. 16-6). For stimulation in the low back and lower extremities, the electrode is initially positioned 2 to 3 mm from the midline on the same side as the patient's pain between the T8 and T10 vertebral levels (Fig. 16-7). Final electrode position is attained by connecting the electrode with an external impulse generator and asking the patient where the pattern of stimulation is felt. In general, cephalad advancement will result in stimulation higher in the extremity and caudad movement will lead to stimulation lower in the extremity. However, if the lead is angled even slightly from medial to lateral, the pattern of stimulation may change less predictably with movement of the electrode (e.g., cephalad advancement can lead to stimulation lower in the extremity under these circumstances). Final electrode position should be recorded using radiography so a permanent lead can be placed in the same position (see Fig. 16-7). For trial stimulation, the needle is then removed, the electrode is secured to the back, and a sterile occlusive dressing is applied (Fig. 16-8). The patient is instructed in the use of the external pulse generator and scheduled to

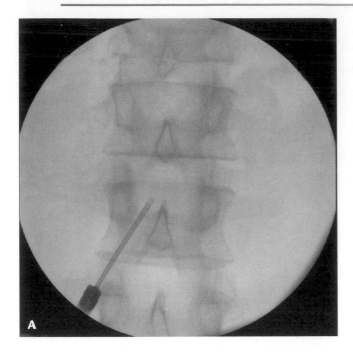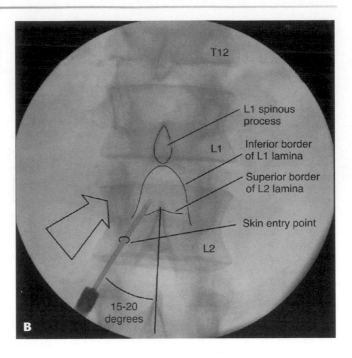

Figure 16-2.
Anterior-Posterior radiograph of initial epidural needle placement for insertion of an epidural spinal cord stimulation electrode. **A:** The c-arm must be carefully aligned to ensure there is no rotation, with the spinous processes aligned in the midline, midway between the vertebral pedicles. The skin entry point for the epidural needle is placed just lateral to the inferior margin of the spinous process that borders the inferior aspect of the interspace to be entered (typically L1/L2 for lower-extremity stimulation and C7/T1 for upper-extremity stimulation). The needle should enter the interspace well below the lamina of the vertebra bordering the superior aspect of the interspace and just to the left or right of midline on the side where you are attempting to advance the electrode. **B:** Labeled image.

return in 5 to 7 days for assessment of his or her response and removal of the trial lead.

During permanent implantation, the procedure for initial lead placement is identical to that for trial stimulation. Once final lead position is attained and the optimal pattern of stimulation is confirmed, the lead must be secured, a pocket for the impulse generator must be created, and the lead tunneled beneath the skin to connect to the impulse generator. Following initial lead placement, the epidural needle is withdrawn slightly (~1 to 2 cm) but left in place around the lead within the subcutaneous tissues to protect the lead during the subsequent incision and dissection. A 5- to 8-cm incision parallel to the axis of the spine is extended from cephalad to caudad to the needle, extending directly through the needle's skin entry point (Fig. 16-9). The subcutaneous tissues are divided using blunt dissection until the lumbar paraspinous fascia is visible surrounding the needle shaft. The stylette is then removed from the lead, and the needle is withdrawn, using care not to dislodge the electrode (Fig. 16-10). The lead is then secured to the paraspinous fascia using a specific anchoring device supplied by the manufacturer (Fig. 16-11).

If lead placement has been carried out in the prone position and the impulse generator is to be placed in the abdominal wall, the lead must be coiled beneath the skin, the paraspinous incision temporarily closed using staples, and a sterile occlusive dressing applied. The sterile drapes are then removed, and the patient is repositioned in the lateral decubitus position with the side where the abdominal pocket will lie upward. After repeat preparation of the skin and application of sterile drapes, attention is turned to creating the pocket within the patient's abdominal wall or overlying the buttock (when the impulse generator is placed over the buttock, this site is included in the initial skin preparation and draping). An 8- to 10-cm transverse incision is made along the previously marked line and a subcutaneous pocket is created using blunt dissection (Fig. 16-12). The pocket should always be created caudad to the incision; if the pocket is placed cephalad to the incision, the weight of the impulse generator on the suture line is likely to cause wound dehiscence. In many patients, the blunt dissection can be accomplished using gentle but firm pressure with the fingers. It is simpler and less traumatic to use a small pair of surgical scissors to perform the blunt dissection using

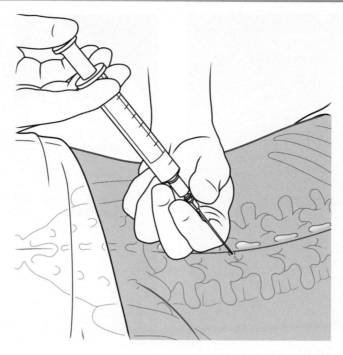

Figure 16-3.
Localization of the epidural space using a loss-of-resistance (LOR) technique. The long and open bevel of the modified Touhy needle used for epidural spinal cord stimulator lead placement rarely yields the clear LOR practitioners are accustomed to when using standard-size epidural needles. One method that can reduce the incidence of false LOR is to advance the epidural needle under fluoroscopic guidance and seat the tip on the superior margin of the lamina that borders the inferior aspect of the interspace to be entered. The area is then bathed with a small amount of local anesthetic to reduce discomfort, and the needle is "walked" over the lamina and into the interlaminar space. Once over the edge of lamina, the needle will enter the ligamentum flavum, and LOR is used during the last few millimeters of needle advancement to identify the epidural space.

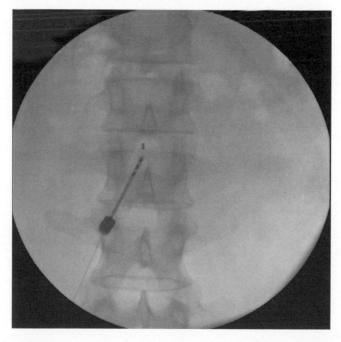

Figure 16-4.
Anterior-Posterior radiograph of epidural needle in final position with the epidural spinal cord stimulation electrode exiting the needle to enter the epidural space. The electrode should be advanced just a few millimeters from the midline to the side where it is to be placed for stimulation.

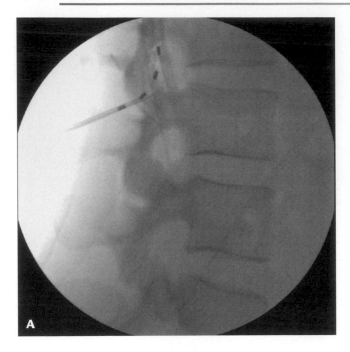
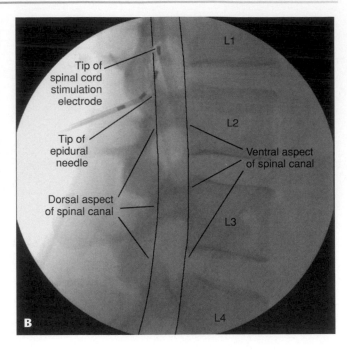

Figure 16-5.
Lateral radiograph of the epidural needle in final position and the spinal cord stimulation electrode exiting the needle to traverse along the dorsal aspect of the epidural space. **A:** If the electrode deviates too far from midline during advancement, its can easily pass around the lateral aspect of the dural sac and course superiorly along the ventral aspect of the epidural space. Ventral electrode placement should be suspected if the patient reports torso stimulation at very low amplitude and can be easily confirmed using lateral radiography. **B:** Labeled image.

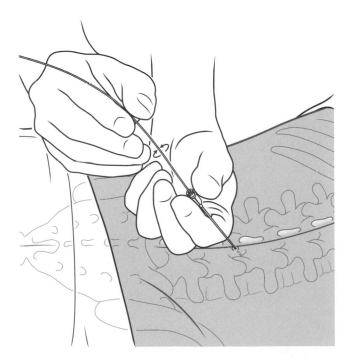

Figure 16-6.
Technique for advancing the epidural spinal cord stimulation electrode. The electrode contains a wire stylette that has a slight angulation at the distal tip. The electrode can be directed medially or laterally as it is advanced under fluoroscopic guidance by using a slight twisting motion on the proximal electrode that changes the direction of the tip.

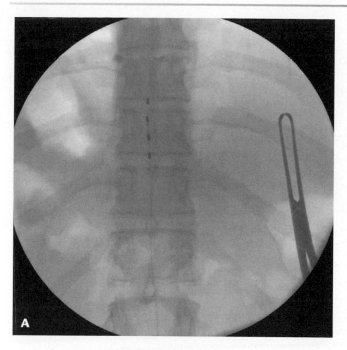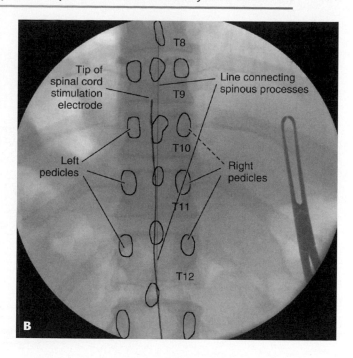

Figure 16-7.
Anterior-Posterior radiograph of the epidural spinal cord stimulation electrode in final position for stimulation of the left lower extremity. **A:** The tip of the electrode is adjacent to the inferior vertebral end plate of T9. A line connecting the spinous processes corresponds to the midline. Note that the lead lies just to the left of midline and has a slight medial-lateral angulation. Optimally, the electrode's course should be parallel to midline so any migration is most likely to move adjacent electrodes into similar positions to one another. **B:** Labeled image.

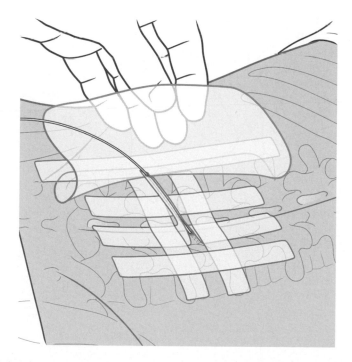

Figure 16-8.
Lead anchor and dressing for temporary lead placement. Sterile bandage strips are placed along the course of the electrode as it exits the skin and then criss-crossed at the base of the electrode to anchor it firmly in place. A sterile occlusive dressing is then applied.

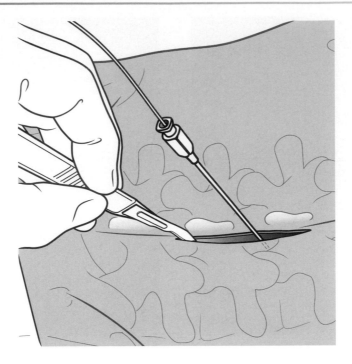

Figure 16-9.
Paraspinous incision. A 5- to 8-cm incision is made through the skin and subcutaneous tissues in a cephalad-caudad direction parallel to midline and to include the needle exit site in the middle of the incision. The needle is left in place around the electrode to protect it from damage during incision and dissection. Blunt dissection is used to divide the subcutaneous tissues and expose the paraspinous fascia.

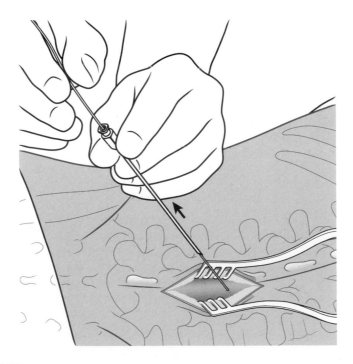

Figure 16-10.
Epidural needle removal. Once the prespinous fascia has been exposed, the stylette and needle are removed, using care not to dislodge the epidural electrode.

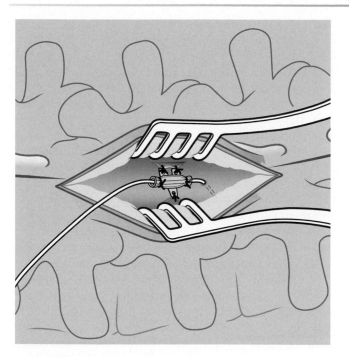

Figure 16-11.
Using a lead anchor supplied by the manufacturer, the electrode is secured to the paraspinous fascia. Once the anchor has been positioned over the electrode, separate sutures should be first placed circumferentially around the anchor and tightened securely so the anchor is firmly in place around the electrode. The anchor is then sutured to the fascia. Attempts to fasten the anchor to the fascia and the lead with a single set of sutures inevitably lead to a loose anchor and increase the likelihood of lead migration.

repeated opening (*not closing or cutting*) motions. After creating the pocket, the impulse generator is placed in the pocket to ensure the pocket is large enough. The impulse generator should fit completely within the pocket without any part of the device extending into the incision. With the device in place, the wound margins must fall into close apposition. There should be no tension on the sutures during closure of the incision or the wound is more likely to dehisce.

After the pocket creation is completed, a tunneling device is extended within the subcutaneous tissues between the paraspinous incision and the pocket (Fig. 16-13). The electrode is then advanced through the tunnel (tunneling devices vary and are specific to each manufacturer). The means with which the electrode is connected to the impulse generator also varies by manufacturer; some devices use a lead extension that connects the impulse generator and the lead, whereas others use a one-piece lead that is connected directly to the impulse generator. After tunneling, the lead and/or lead extension is connected with the impulse generator. Any excess lead is coiled and placed behind the impulse generator within the pocket (Fig. 16-14). This loop allows for patient movement without placing tension on the distal electrode and causing it to be pulled from the epidural space. The skin incisions are then closed in two

layers: a series of interrupted subcutaneous sutures to securely close the fascia overlying the impulse generator within the pocket, and the electrode over the paraspinous fascia followed by a skin closure using suture or staples (Fig. 16-15). Alternately, according to patient preference, the impulse generator can be placed in a pocket overlying the buttock, using care to remain well below the superior margins of the iliac crest (Fig. 16-16).

Complications

Bleeding and infection are risks inherent to all open surgical procedures. Bleeding within the impulse generator pocket can lead to a hematoma surrounding the generator that may require surgical drainage. Bleeding along the subcutaneous tunneling track often causes significant bruising in the region but rarely requires treatment. Similar to other neuraxial techniques, bleeding within the epidural space can lead to significant neural compression. Signs of infection within the impulse generator pocket typically occur within 10 to 14 days following implantation but may occur at any time. Some practitioners have reported successful treatment of superficial infections of the incision overlying the pocket with oral antibiotics aimed at the offending

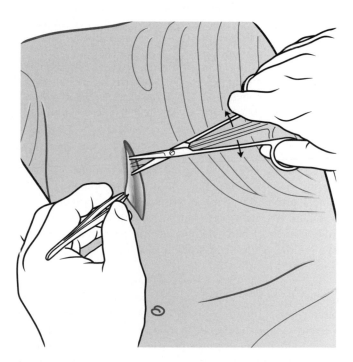

Figure 16-12.
Creation of a subcutaneous pocket for the implanted pulse generator. An 8- to 10-cm transverse incision is created just below the costal margin, using care to avoid placement too lateral. The skin is incised using a sharp scalpel, and the subcutaneous pocket is then created using blunt dissection (using surgical scissors in an opening rather than a closing or cutting motion works effectively).

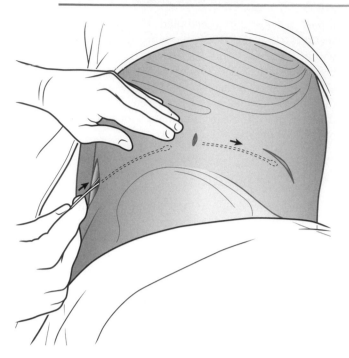

Figure 16-13.
Subcutaneous tunneling of the electrode. Using the device provided by the manufacturer, a subcutaneous tunnel is created, and the electrode is passed from paraspinous region to the pocket. Care must be taken to continuously palpate the tip of the tunneling device as it is being advanced to ensure the depth of the subcutaneous track is neither too deep nor too shallow. Excess depth can lead to entry into the abdominal cavity, whereas too shallow of a tunnel can lead to skin perforation or visible puckering of the skin along the subcutaneous track. In large patients, the tunneling often requires two segments; the first segment between the paravertebral incision and a small transverse incision in the mid-axillary line, and a second segment from the mid-axillary line to the abdominal pocket.

organism and close observation alone. However, infections within the pocket or along the lead's subcutaneous course almost universally require removal of all implanted hardware and treatment with parenteral antibiotics to eradicate infection. Lead and deep tissue infections can extend to involve the neuraxis and result in epidural abscess formation and/or meningitis.

There is a significant risk of dural puncture during initial localization of the epidural space using the LOR technique. The epidural needle used for electrode placement is a Tuohy needle that has been modified by extending the orifice to allow the electrode to pass easily. This long bevel often results in equivocal LOR. It is not uncommon to have minimal resistance to injection along the entire course of needle placement. To minimize the risk of dural puncture, the needle tip can be advanced under fluoroscopic guidance and first seated on the margin of the vertebral lamina (using care to place additional local anesthetic during advancement). In this way, the depth of the lamina is certain, and the needle need only be advanced a small distance over the lam-

ina, through the ligamentum flavum, and into the epidural space. LOR is used only during the final few millimeters of needle advancement over the lamina. If dural puncture does occur, there is no clear consensus on how to proceed. Some practitioners will abandon the lead placement and allow 1 to 2 weeks before reattempting placement. This approach allows the practitioner to watch and treat postdural puncture headache, which is nearly certain to occur. Other practitioners will proceed with lead placement through a more cephalad interspace. If postdural puncture headache ensues and fails conservative treatment, epidural blood patch is then placed at the level of the dural puncture. Spinal cord and nerve root injury during initial lead placement have been reported. Placing the epidural needle and lead in the awake, lightly sedated patient able to report paresthesiae should minimize the risk of direct neural injury.

The most frequent complication following spinal cord stimulator placement is lead migration. The first line of defense is to ensure the lead is firmly secured to the paraspinous fascia. Suturing the lead to loose subcutaneous tissue or fat is not adequate. Postoperatively, the patient must be clearly instructed to avoid bending and twisting at the waist (lumbar leads) or bending and twisting the neck (cervical leads) for at least 4 weeks after lead placement. Placing a soft cervical collar on those who have had a cervical lead placed provides a ready reminder to avoid movement. Lead fracture may also occur, often months or years

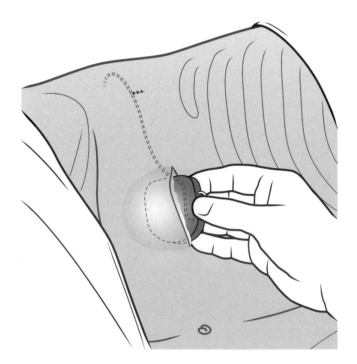

Figure 16-14.
Placement of the implanted pulse generator into the subcutaneous pocket. Any excess lead is coiled behind the impulse generator, and care is used to ensure the pocket is large enough to prevent any tension on the margins of the incision. The impulse generator and lead should fit well inferior to the incision so risk of damage is minimized at the time of subsequent operation for battery change.

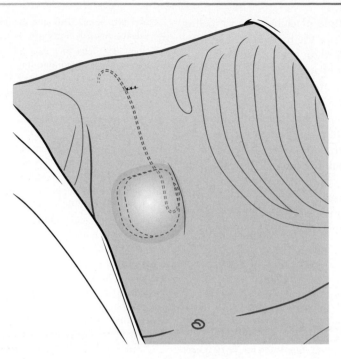

Figure 16-15.
Wound closure. The pocket is closed in two separate suture layers. The subcutaneous tissues are closed over the impulse generator and the lead in the paraspinous region, using interrupted, absorbable suture followed by a separate skin closure using staples or sutures (simple interrupted or running subcuticular for better cosmesis).

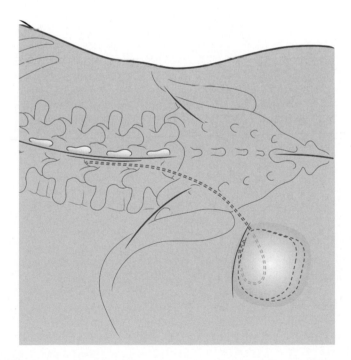

Figure 16-16.
Alternate pocket location over the buttock. Some practitioners and patients prefer to place the implanted pulse generator over the buttock. This allows for the entire implant procedure to be carried out in the prone position. Care should be used to ensure the pocket is well below the bony margins of the iliac crest. Placement too near the iliac crest can lead to marked discomfort on sitting as the impulse generator is forced against the bone.

after placement. Avoiding midline placement or tunneling the lead across midline will reduce the incidence of fracture caused by compression of the lead on bone. Lead fracture is signaled by a sudden loss of stimulation and is diagnosed by checking lead impedance using the spinal cord stimulator programmer.

Wound dehiscence and impulse generator migration are infrequent problems. Ensuring the size of the pocket is sufficient to prevent tension on the suture line at the time of wound closure is essential to minimize the risk of dehiscence.

Subcutaneous collection of fluid surrounding the impulse generator (seroma formation) can be problematic and typically follows generator replacement. Percutaneous drainage of the sterile fluid collection is often successful in resolving the problem.

SUGGESTED READINGS

Augustinsson LE. Spinal cord stimulation in peripheral vascular disease and angina pectoris. *J Neurosurg Sci.* 2003;47(Suppl 1):37–40.

Cameron T. Safety and efficacy of spinal cord stimulation for the treatment of chronic pain: a 20-year literature review. *J Neurosurg.* 2004;100 (3 Suppl):254–267.

Carter ML. Spinal cord stimulation in chronic pain: a review of the evidence. *Anaesth Intensive Care.* 2004;32:11–21.

Grabow TS, Tella PK, Raja SN. Spinal cord stimulation for complex regional pain syndrome: an evidence-based medicine review of the literature. *Clin J Pain.* 2003;19:371–383.

Kemler MA, De Vet HC, Barendse GA et al. The effect of spinal cord stimulation in patients with chronic reflex sympathetic dystrophy: two years' follow-up of the randomized controlled trial. *Ann Neurol.* 2004;55: 13–18.

Oakley JC. Spinal cord stimulation: patient selection, technique, and outcomes. *Neurosurg Clin N Am.* 2003;14:365–380, vi.

Ohnmeiss DD, Rashbaum RF. Patient satisfaction with spinal cord stimulation for predominant complaints of chronic, intractable low back pain. *Spine J.* 2001;1:358–363.

Quigley DG, Arnold J, Eldridge PR et al. Long-term outcome of spinal cord stimulation and hardware complications. *Stereotact Funct Neurosurg.* 2003;81:50–56.

Simpson BA. Spinal-cord stimulation for reflex sympathetic dystrophy. *Lancet Neurol.* 2004;3:142.

Taylor RS, Taylor RJ, Van Buyten JP et al. The cost effectiveness of spinal cord stimulation in the treatment of pain: a systematic review of the literature. *J Pain Symptom Manage.* 2004;27:370–378.

Turner JA, Loeser JD, Deyo RA et al. Spinal cord stimulation for patients with failed back surgery syndrome or complex regional pain syndrome: a systematic review of effectiveness and complications. *Pain.* 2004;108: 137–147.

Index